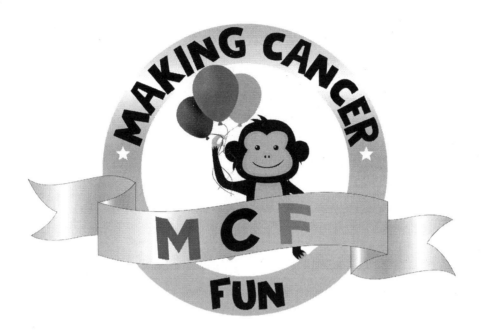

a PaRent's Guide

taRa GeRaGHtY

Making Cancer Fun: A Parent's Guide by Tara Geraghty

Published by Minipoka Publishing PO BOX 420 Franklin Lakes NJ 07417

© 2016 Minipoka Publishing a Division of Pink Heart Inc.

For information about special discounts available for bulk purchases, sales promotions, fund-raising and educational needs, contact Minipoka Publishing at 1-201-800-4179 or pinkheartinc@mail.com

Special Thanks to Consultant & Editor Laura Gingberg and
Book Designer Cattani Creative LLC. www.cattanicreative.com

ISBN-13:978-0578425870

ISBN-10:0578425874

This book is dedicated to all the Miracle Kids
we are ever lucky enough to meet.

Your purchase makes a difference.

A percentage of this book's profits are donated to non-profits
that make cancer fun for children in honor of John Catt,
a man who spent his life Making Cancer Fun for Kids.

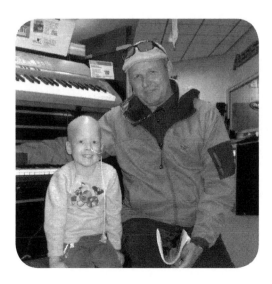

ENDORSEMENTS

"As an Oncology/Bone Marrow Transplant Nurse for the last 10 years, I have seen patients and families experience the diagnosis of cancer in many different ways. Tara and Emily were truly unique. I have no doubt in my mind that Emily's success in healing and remaining cancer free are due to the way Tara chose to approach this disease and treatment. Making Cancer Fun *is something I would recommend to any family facing the challenges of this devastating disease. Even if the outcome is not the same as Emily's, this book will help families and patients to make the absolute most out of a debilitating situation. This book is brilliant!!"*

 —Nanette Cavanaugh, RN
  Banner Desert Medical Center - Oncology

"It took a lot of strength and courage for Tara to revisit the emotions attached to this traumatic time. I am so grateful that she did. This book will change the way families face cancer and disease going forward. I watched in awe as Emily laughed and had fun through the most challenging and difficult time I could ever imagine a child experiencing. Tara and Emily's positive attitude turned their worst nightmare into an incredible display of perseverance, courage, and even joy. I've been an Oncology nurse and patient advocate for 12 years. Making Cancer Fun *is the most valuable tool I've seen throughout my nursing career. This book will empower families to gain control over a terrifying situation the best way they can. These tools will enable parent's ability to bring smiles to their loved ones and create beautiful memories that will last a lifetime. Tara has presented us with an incredible gift and I encourage ALL patients and families who are fighting illness to read this book!"*

 —Christine Frodella RN, OCN
  Oncology Nurse Navigator
  Heme Malignancy and Bone Marrow Transplant Program
  University of Colorado Hospital

"Cancer Fun!?! This was my first thought when I heard the name of this book. Then, I remembered who I was dealing with! Of all the families, Emily's mom was determined to make this time the best she could for her 'Miracle Child.' I remember being in an elevator with other people, taking Emily somewhere, and Tara had a hand puppet that was talking to people riding with us. Some parents wouldn't have done this for embarrassment to themselves. Tara was selfless when it

came to Em, if it made Emily smile, Tara would do it. I saw that parent later in the day and they asked me if 'the mom' was 'okay'. I had to laugh and say, 'Yes, she is just trying to make her daughter laugh.' Reading this book, has brought me back to those days and how much effort Tara put into making sure Emily had 'fun' in the scary world of cancer. Sharing her experience with actual events and providing interactive ideas, can help kids of all ages. As Oncology nurses, we meet people on their worst day, and this book helps to bring some insight and sunshine into the darkest of days."

—Melissa L. Vickers, Pediatric RN, BSN

"Cancer completely changes families; sometimes families flourish and sometimes families fall apart. Families who can find joy, reasons to have gratitude and a few ways to have fun are so much more likely to flourish! Tara brings so many practical and tangible ideas to the table on how to make the awful reality of cancer a little more manageable by celebrating the little (or big) successes! This book will be a great resource to new families as they begin their journey in the kid cancer club."

—Jocelyn Zauche MS, CPNP-PC, FNP-BC, CPHON

"Tara Geraghty has mastered the art of positivity in the face of darkness. This is the ultimate survival guide for a family facing what is undoubtedly the ugliest and scariest times of their lives. This survival guide will provide you with the tools needed to stay strong as a family unit—no matter the surrounding dynamics of your own personal situation. Sharing in Tara and Em's journey will surely bring you one step closer to experiencing an inner peace and allow your family to find a way to say 'LIFE IS GOOD' in a very difficult time."

—Jennifer A. Giordano RN-BC
Saint Peters University Hospital
Camp Quality New Jersey

ACKNOWLEDGMENTS

Thank you to all the people who believed that what we did during Emily's cancer treatment was different and valuable enough to share with others. Thank you to Nannette, Jocelyn, Melissa, Dr. Jennifer Bruny, Anna, Dr. Ben, Dr. Matthew, Dr. Brian, and Dr. Karen Fay for your medical brilliance and for taking care of my Miracle Baby. I could never have enough thank yous to all my friends who loved on me and Emily. Thank you to my Mary Kay family for doing fundraisers, to Shana Earp for bringing Santa, to Yvette for bringing Mother Christmas. Thank you to Bethany and John Skorich for being our Colorado family. Your prayers matter more than you will ever know. Thank you to Erin Rose, Jaime W. & Irene S. for helping me feel normal and for being my sisters by love. Thank you Paul P. for letting me just be me around you. Thank you to Debbie S. for not charging me for all the therapy you've given me and for believing in me when I didn't. Thank you Cory J. for changing my life in one day with your Christmas gift. Thank you to Jordyn H. for sitting with me during Emily's 8-hour tumor removal surgery. Thank you Danielle B., Meredith G., and Rebecca M. who accept me just for me. Thank you to my Cousin Christine for going into Oncology and not letting me stay in the ER room when they cut Emily open that first night. Thank you to my Aunt Janet, who is also my Godmother, and sometimes a second mother when it comes to advice. Thank you to my sister Laura, my brothers Lonnie and Jamie, and my SIL Caroline: You had no choice; you had to love Emily because you are her family. Thank you to my Dad for taking care of us. Thank you to my Mom for giving up your life, moving across the country, and sleeping in a hospital chair for a year. Thank you to Lynn G., Barbara C., and Dorothy M. for being family by love. Thank you to Rebekah Welch because without your encouragement to record my story this may have never been shared. Thank you to Heather L. and Laura G. for taking my "word vomit" and teaching me what a book is. Thank you Emily Grace, you are my gift from God and the one person I love more than anyone in this world and the biggest blessing in my life. I believe I was created to be your mom. I love you, my miracle baby. Always remember, God has a plan for YOU. He has protected and guided you since the day you were born. I can't wait to see the woman you will choose to become.

♥ Mommy .

FOREWORD

I've never understood how families do it. I tell people their child has cancer, and I just know they must feel the world crashing in on them. While parents inevitably have instincts to fight and protect, families have varying degrees of success at navigating the psychological and emotional battle cancer wages on them. As a medical provider, I feel like I have not always had great insight into what can make a difference in that battle.

Over the years, I have seen children and families have various responses during their cancer fight. Some are outward fighters; others fight internally. Most parents grapple with some need for control in a situation where so many things are uncontrollable. Some kids get more mature, while others regress.

I am delighted that Tara and Emily have chosen to share their very personal take on this journey. They took control of the fight rather than letting the massiveness of the battle overwhelm them. Tara also actively empowered Emily to take charge of her own battle, even at age 3. They are living proof that cancer may take things from you, but it can't take away your spirit or the essence of who you are. Clearly, stupid cancer messed with the wrong kid.

The lessons in this book are not just for parents, but for medical providers as well. If you are a doctor, a nurse, advanced practice provider, child life specialist, physical therapist, etc., and your practice touches the lives of children with cancer (or more appropriately, children with cancer touch your life), then this book will teach you things.

One of the main pearls of wisdom I gained from this book is to be intentional with your choices. As a parent, are you going to change your discipline style? As a family, how are you going to deal with painful things that are inevitable? As medical professionals or as part of a support system, how are we going to deal with difficult conversations?

Just recently, I met a family whose son had just been diagnosed with leukemia. They were still reeling from the initial shock while I was trying to tell them about the port we needed to implant. Mom was struggling with this "thing" we needed to put in her child and with how to tell her child about it. In just a brief conversation, I suggested calling the port his "champion" and thinking of it as one of his weapons in his battle against cancer, which is something I learned from Tara. I saw a spark in the mom's eyes: the idea of flipping this "thing" into something positive could work for them.

I can tell families we have the best treatment and the smartest team, but I can't tell a family how to fight, how to protect their child, and how to empower their child, but I believe this book is a great introduction to the miracle mentality.

Jennifer Bruny, MD
Director of Surgical Oncology
Children's Hospital Colorado
Proud Miracle Kid Sidekick

TABLE OF CONTENTS

YOUR iNitiation into CLUB Cancer

Welcome to Orientation

Welcome to the club. Club Cancer. It's an initiation I never wanted, and I know you don't want it either. I'm sorry I am the one to welcome you. It's actually a secret club that no one wants membership to, but now we're part of it, forever. If you are like me, you probably want to run and hide, and you probably are still secretly hoping this is all a nightmare you will wake up from any minute. I get it. I remember my initiation. It was back in November 2009 when my 3½ year old, Emily Grace, was diagnosed with High Risk Stage 4 Neruoblastoma (a sticky tumor). I had to keep checking the spelling as I was trying to Google it because I didn't know how to say it, much less spell it. I physically felt ill the first time I saw a bald kid in "real life."

I don't know the journey that led you here, to the club, or to this book, but if you are now a "cancer parent," we are forever bonded. We share a secret bond that other parents, fortunately, will never understand. If I sat across from you, looked you in the eyes, I would know, and you would know, that we understand each other. We've seen (or are currently facing) the other side of darkness. We now value every second with our children in a way most parents will never have the gift of appreciating. We know the difference in celebrating birthdays, holidays, and milestones that the rest of the world doesn't. Each time we hear of a new child diagnosed with cancer—whether it's a year, five years, ten years, or possibly a lifetime from now, we will have that deep, profound understanding of what that parent is initially going through: the shock, the anger, the frustration, the guilt, the tears, the fears, the stress, the overwhelmingness, and the sometimes wanting to just sit on the bottom of the shower floor, put our hands on our faces and cry. The helplessness.

> "If you have struggled through something, and survived, you should then help those who are still struggling.
>
> Brendon Burchard, author of _The Millionaire Messenger_"

It's my hope that this book will help you regain your hope and your control and that it will help change the way your child will face cancer.

When I look back over my life B.C. (before cancer) I think God was preparing me for Emily's cancer. For a long time I took for granted that my unique life experiences and background meant that when she was diagnosed I would approach it differently than most families. I just figured everyone did what we did—throw a party. I mean, after all, one of my first professional jobs after college was touring with a children's theater company. Maybe my years of improvisation, learning how to think and speak on my feet while working with improv teachers from around the country, prepared me for cancer. Or maybe it was my 10+ years in the direct sales industry with a company that constantly recognized achievements and turned everything into a party, that prepared me to make cancer fun. I'm not sure, but I think those three things and possibly, just maybe, my personality (or stubbornness) gave me a unique perspective.

It's my hope that from reading this book, you will feel empowered and equipped to take control of a situation that feels uncontrollable. Maybe you'll be comforted in knowing there is another parent, me, who "gets" what you are going through. Maybe you'll find an idea you can incorporate into your child's own cancer battle. Or maybe you'll discover hope and light at the end of the tunnel, and that cancer doesn't need to be your whole life, it can just be a season. If any of that resonates with you, then read on.

It wasn't until about half-way through Emily's cancer treatment, when the chaplain from the hospital asked if I would meet with one of her interns and share the fun things we had been doing, that I began to think, "Maybe not everyone approaches cancer the same way?"

She said the energy in our room was "different." Since I had never been in any of the other children's rooms I didn't really understand what she meant by "different." She explained that many times when a family gets the diagnosis of cancer, the dreaded C word, almost instantly everything turns somber. The laughter stops. The fun stops. The terror takes over. Rooms become serious, quiet, and totally focused on the medical intricacy of cancer. Everyone becomes scared and worried. That is understandable, because after all, cancer and your child potentially dying aren't things to joke about or to take lightly. It is easy for the heaviness of cancer to take over as a void of darkness as despair settles in.

Yet, in our room it was apparently different. Opposite really. We made fun of cancer. We found things to laugh about. We joked about it. For a lot of families, I guess I can see how that might seem offensive: How could we joke about something so serious?

For me, if our life for the moment was inside the confines of a hospital room I was going to make it as fun as possible. All the medicine, chemo, and surgeries, while obviously critical, in my mind would be unsuccessful if my daughter's spirit didn't have the will to fight. If she was going to fight to simply be wheeled back into a dark, depressing room filled with sadness and tears, would she fight as hard? I vowed to make her room and her experience so fun that she would fight with everything she had. I wanted her to have something to look forward to each day and to remind her that this was

not for forever, this was just right now, and that right now we would have fun.

Now, maybe you are assuming it was easy for me to make cancer fun simply because my daughter survived. You might try to rationalize that because my child responded well to treatment and lived that it makes sense and that of course Making Cancer Fun was easy, right? After all, I didn't lose my child. My Club Cancer must have had a different membership option.

Guess what? I decided to make cancer fun long before I knew if Emily would live— long before I knew how she would react to treatment, chemotherapy or surgery.

I decided how I would react to her cancer before I knew if she would survive.

I made up my mind from the very beginning that she was going to be victorious. I set my mind on faith and consciously chose to trust and believe that she was going to survive. That was the reality I chose to live in even when no one knew what the outcome was going to be. It wasn't that I made cancer fun after I saw her respond well to treatment. I believe part of why she responded well to treatment is because I made cancer fun! Now Making Cancer Fun has no guarantees, and there was no guarantee my daughter was going to survive no matter how much fun we had, the only choice I had was how I was going to face it, and I chose fun.

What about you? What will you choose? Over the years I have seen so many friends lose their precious children. It's hard because it's not fair. I'm keenly aware I don't love my child more than they loved theirs, and I don't deserve to have my child survive any more or less than anyone else. But I often think, if I had only a few months, a few weeks, a few days, or even just a few hours left with my child how would I want to spend them? It's a sobering thought. Would I want that precious time to be somber and solemn in a hospital room filled with fear and dread, waiting for the end? Or would I want the atmosphere to be fun and silly with giggles, laughter, and love?

I don't know your personal situation, but I often think of the families I know who have children who aren't responding to treatment. It may

be their last days or moments spent here on earth with their precious children. Fleeting moments that will be stolen by death too soon. That's why, in my humble opinion, it's even more important to make cancer fun and to fill those last moments with memories that in our darkest hours of despair will make us smile and laugh remembering the fun we had through the moments of pain. What memories do you want to create?

Being part of Club Cancer changes your perspective. After all, none of us knows what the future's going to hold. Life is said to be short, but for cancer kids, life is sometimes temporary. Making Cancer Fun is about more than just helping children with cancer; it's a metaphor for how we should live our lives every day even outside of the cancer world. How many people get into a car on their way home from work and never make it home? (Statistically, it's 119 a day!) How many freak accidents, heart attacks, or aneurysms happen every day? How many tragedies happen to children with mass shootings in our schools and churches? Life is fragile, and in our hustle and bustle we forget that fact until we are face-to-face with

Your Initiation Into Club Cancer. Welcome to Orientation.

5

the reality of death. Making Cancer Fun reminds us that every moment could potentially be the last memories we are creating with someone. What do we want those memories to be? We need to lighten up, enjoy, be silly, have fun, let our guard down, and giggle a little more every day. We never know when those moments might be our final ones.

So how does one live through something that can only be described as a living nightmare? Something beyond any pain a parent or child should ever have to endure? Losing a child is horrific enough. Losing a child to cancer is like watching the person you love more than yourself be taken over by death slowly, as if the Devil himself were in charge. I'm eternally grateful and humbled that I have never had to endure that level of pain because I know the pain I feel for the children I have seen die is overwhelming enough. I'll never forget the pain I felt watching one of our favorite nurses stand outside her patient's intensive care unit in tears moments after his final breath. Watching her sob I called her over to peek in on my Miracle

Baby sitting in her own hospital bed across the hall to remind her what she does every day does make a difference. Some children do live. My mantra became: if someone is going to live, why not my kid? Why not yours? If Making Cancer Fun is a choice, it's a choice I choose. Will you?

Now I get it, just because we make something fun, just because we have a great attitude, just because we put a smile on when we feel like crying doesn't change the reality of what our children are going to go through. It doesn't change the pain. It doesn't change the worry. It doesn't change the fear. Those are real things

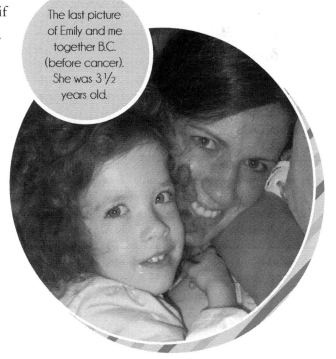

The last picture of Emily and me together B.C. (before cancer). She was 3 ½ years old.

we experience. So, why write "Making Cancer Fun?" Why share these things? I know it's not going to change the facts of our circumstances. I know there are parents who will read this and, within days, lose their children. I wish, more than anything, that writing a book would make cancer go away and sharing, "Hey, this can be fun!" would change things. That if you just make it fun, it won't be so painful, you won't lose your child, they won't suffer and they won't have pain. I would write a thousand books if that were the case.

So what's my hope? My hope is that this book becomes a tool. A place you can go back to for support. A place where you can take an idea, a tip, or an inspiration and make your journey a little easier. To add one more smile, one more giggle, or one more peal of laughter. I hope there's something you find to hold onto, to make the pain and fear little less, and to calm your worries.

I'll share with you tips, techniques, and tools along with a peek into our Making Cancer Fun world. I'll challenge you to think differently about cancer, to think differently about yourself, and to do some things that might make your child roll their eyes (hopefully followed by a giggle or two!) If you're naturally silly, great! If not, this might be a step out of your comfort zone. That's the thing about Club Cancer: you get to choose. You can sit on the sidelines and cry or get in the game and play. I hope you'll find reasons to celebrate and throw a party so that in the end there might be more tears of laughter than tears of pain.

> Being part of Club Cancer can make you stronger or weaker, but you will be changed.

What's one thing you could do today to make your journey a little more fun? One thing you could do today to make your child's day a little brighter, a little sillier? What's one thing you could do right now to laugh about? Don't worry, if you don't know yet, you will by the end of this book! I really believe that if we keep laughing, even in the face of fear, doubt, and pain, while those things may still be there, we will not allow the enemy to steal us of our joy, our peace, or our fun. I hope you'll join me on this journey so that we can try, from this day forward, together to make cancer fun.

Your Initiation Into Club Cancer. Welcome to Orientation.

7

SOME 2017 STATS ABOUT YOUR MEMBERSHIP TO CLUB CANCER...You're Not Alone.

- Every 2 minutes a child is diagnosed with cancer.
  STBALDWICKS.ORG

- 1 in 320 children will be diagnosed with cancer before the age of 20.
  CURESEARCH.ORG

- The average age of children diagnosed is 6.
  CURESEARCH.ORG

- More than 40,000 children undergo treatment for cancer each year.
  CURESEARCH.ORG

- There are approximately 375,000 adult survivors of children's cancer in the United States. That equates to 1 in 530 adults ages 20 to 39.
  CURESEARCH.ORG

- Childhood cancer does not discriminate and spares no child based on ethnic background, socio-economic class, or geographic location.
  CURESEARCH.ORG

YOUR NEW JOB: CANCER FUN-MAKER

Think On Your Feet & Think Like a Kid

"So yeah, that's not supposed to be there," the Emergency Room X-Ray tech explained as he showed me my daughter's CAT scan results of her stomach. He pointed to a large white circle that looked about the size of a baseball to me.

"Why, what is it?" I asked.

"Um, I'm not the person who can tell you," he responded.

"Ok…so who can?" I asked impatiently.

"They're sending someone down from Oncology," he said. In 2009, naive, blissful, ignorant little me didn't know what the word oncology meant. My mother did, though, and she turned white as he spoke. A little while later I found myself in a parent consult room while a doctor explained they thought my daughter had cancer. They were pretty sure it was neuroblastoma, and they were biopsying the tumor to confirm. Honestly, looking back it's like bits and pieces of a movie I've seen, know the story to, but somehow fade all together and don't really remember. We all get to the same place though: the final cancer diagnosis. Most parents I talk to knew something was wrong. Some hadn't even been like us, back and forth multiple times to multiple doctors. But cancer was never anything that crossed anybody's mind. Who thinks their kid's stomachache is cancer? (Okay, truth be told it was a long time post-cancer before Emily could have a stomachache, an earache, or a headache without me thinking, "Dear God, please don't let it be cancer again.")

The next morning as I sat in the Intensive Care Unit with my 3-year-old hooked up to IVs, lines, beeping things, and a large chest tube they surgically implanted the night before, I had a lot of explaining to do. When it was my first day on my new job as a full-time cancer fun maker, I had no idea where to even begin. Maybe without ever knowing it, all those years of studying improv were for moments just like this. See, often during cancer, a doctor will walk into your room, tell you something about your child's

> **Where there is laughter, there is life.**
>
> *The Anti-Cancer Club*

patient care, and then you'll have to turn around and explain it in a way a little mind can comprehend. Now, I don't know about you, but I don't have a medical background. Often I would still be trying to wrap my head around what they said, never mind being able to explain it to my kid.

So I'm going to give you a crash course in Improv 101. Ready? It's simple. It's called, "Yes, and…" Yup, that's the number one rule in improv. Whatever your partner says, you agree with and then add something. If you're on stage and your partner says, "Isn't it a beautiful day here on Mars?" You can't say, "No dummy we're in California. No one has ever been to Mars!" You have to say, "Why YES, today is beautiful on Mars, AND I love vacationing here." You start to add to the scene. Not only do you agree you are on Mars, but now you're helping build the scene and explaining you are on vacation. Get it?

So How does that Make cancer fun? Let Me explain.

Remember that first day when Emily woke up with a chest tube sticking out of her left side? Well, when the doctors first showed me her lung X-rays all I could see was white. Her entire lung was white on one whole

side and then about halfway down the other side. It was so white I wouldn't have even known it was a lung if they didn't tell me what I was looking at!

They explained to me that I was looking at fluid that had filled up and around her lungs. She had a pleural effusion, and that was why they had to do emergency surgery. They needed to cut her open, drain out as much fluid as they could, and put in a chest tube.

Now, I had the awkward task of explaining to a 3-year-old what had just happened. I mean how do you explain a tumor? A chest tube? Fluid flowing out of your lungs? So, YES there is fluid coming out of your lungs, AND it is coconut juice. I know….coconut juice. In my defense it was white and it did look like coconut juice to me, and it was the first thing that popped into my head. So embracing my years of improvisational training, I just went with it.

I told her that somehow her lungs had filled up with coconut juice, and the doctors needed to get the coconut juice out. I explained that they needed to put a tube in her chest to take out the coconut juice.

In retrospect, had I realized that the fluid was going to come out laced with blood, looking red and various shades of pink, I probably would have used the term "fruit punch" instead, but I hadn't seen the actual fluid yet, I only saw the white X-ray, which, in my mind, looked like coconut juice. Later on, she did ask me why the coconut juice was red, and I never really had a solid answer. We just started referring to it as coconut juice, and it stuck. She had that chest tube for a long time! For almost two months she was hooked up to a little box that would bubble and sounded like a fish tank. I would go to sleep every night, listening to that fish tank-like sound. I remember when she finally got rid of her chest tube, it was difficult to sleep without that bubbling aquarium sound lulling in the background.

When the nurses would come in at night to change out the box we would say they were coming to change out the coconut juice. One time, she looked at me with all seriousness and asked, "Mommy, how did all that coconut juice get in me? I don't remember drinking any coconut juice?" I told her I didn't know, but somehow that coconut juice had snuck into her.

One time she also asked me, "Where do they take the coconut juice?" Again, this is where I had to think on my feet. So, YES they take your coconut juice, AND they give it to the monkeys who live on top of the hospital and like to eat coconuts.

In disbelief she said, "What? There are monkeys on top of the hospital?" I told her yes, there were monkeys that lived on the top floor of the hospital, and they needed to have something to eat, and so they would take all the coconut juice that kids have and send it upstairs to the monkeys. I guess in my mind I pictured a palm tree with a coconut, and a monkey hanging off of it. Then we would talk about the monkeys with their coconut juice, and how much coconut juice they were getting today, and whether or not they liked the coconut juice or what it must taste like.

I remember when she finally got her chest tube out, and there was no more coconut juice. We talked about how sad the monkeys were going to be that they didn't have anything to drink anymore! They were going to have to find another kid to get coconut juice from since they couldn't get any more from her because, after all, she was kicking cancer's butt!

Fun Factor

What is a procedure your child needs to do?

_____

What is the reason why? *(This is your YES!)*

_____

_____

_____

What does it make you think of?

_____

_____

What image pops into your mind? *An animal? A color? A place? A song?*

_____

_____

If you had to draw a picture of it what would you draw?

What could be fun or silly about it? *(This is your AND!)*

_____

_____

_____

Fun Factor

Why does your kid think he or she needs to have this procedure done?

_____

_____

_____

_____

What does the procedure look like to your kid?

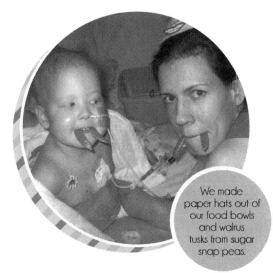

THE BOTTOM LINE

How Silly Can You Make it?

We made paper hats out of our food bowls and walrus tusks from sugar snap peas.

A Peek Into Our World...Baldness, Curls, and Crying

I'll never forget sitting in the car when Emily's doctor called me to tell me that it was confirmed. Her tumor was exactly what they anticipated...high-risk Stage IV cancer. In some ways, it was a relief to finally have an answer. At least then we could start moving forward, even if it was the worst-case scenario. Briefly, the doctor explained her medical team would get together with me to explain her treatment, which would involve chemotherapy, removing the tumor, a bone marrow transplant, radiation, and potentially some biotherapy. I had a few questions, but it was the last one that will always stay etched in my memory. Picture me pulled over in the car, sitting next to my mom. The last question I asked was my most burning: "I know this is a silly question, in light of what you just told me, but will she lose her hair?" In the back

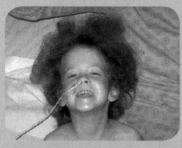

The night we finally cut Emily's hair short.

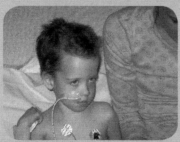

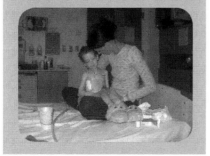

of my mind, I thought, this woman just told me my child has Stage IV cancer, and my concern is whether or not she's going to lose her hair? But I had to know, would she lose her hair? Her doctor said, "Yes, she will lose her hair." I replied, "I know, I know, it's a silly question." She said, "It's not a silly question. It's the outward sign of the disease."

When Emily's hair started falling out, we cut it really short. I was actually going to cut my hair with her, but the girl who did my hair always seemed to have a cold and could never come to the floor, which was kept on germ-free lock down. So, as her hair started falling out we just started cutting it shorter. And then a little shorter. I could never bring myself to fully shave her head. I remember the night we cropped it super short. I sat on her bed with her in my lap, cutting away. Emily sat there, and she said, "Mommy, can I have a piece?" She took a long piece of hair and sat there brushing it. My heart broke.

That night as I crawled into bed, I sobbed and sobbed, and sobbed some more. Quietly, of course, so Emily couldn't hear me across the room. Until I heard a little voice lean over the edge of her bed, and say, "Mommy, why are you crying? I'm still right here." In that moment, I knew God spoke to me through her. Saying, "Don't cry; she's right here. It's just hair. She's still here. And she'll stay here." It was one of those moments I remember in my memory like a picture. I remember that feeling. I remember that little voice. I remember that sense of peace, that assurance, the Spirit speaking directly to me through my 3-year-old and saying, "It will be okay."

Emily didn't like her hair before cancer. It was crazy curly with Shirley Temple ringlets all over her little head. And while people always commented on what incredible hair she had, for a little girl that needed her hair brushed, washed, and detangled, gorgeous curls were not fun. Especially washing through those tangles of curls, which seemed like a nightmare. Now in retrospect some tangles don't seem so "nightmarish" after all. When her hair started falling out, she wanted to know, "Why? Why is my hair falling out?" I told her that God figured if she had to deal with cancer, and go through all that, then she wasn't going to have to wash her hair and comb through knots too. It actually made her quite pleased to have her hair fall out. No more washing her hair. No more cutting through tangles. I remember when her hair started growing back, she was about 5-years-old and I had to actually buy shampoo for her. I said, "Em, you're going have to start washing your hair again!" She said, "Mom, shave my head! I don't want hair!"

While she was bald, friends would buy her cute headbands, scarves, and hats to wear. Yet Emily never wanted to cover her bald head; she loved to show it off. She was proud of her bald head. And, over time, I began to love her bald head, too. When her hair grew back in, I was surprised how emotional I was. It felt as if she was losing her little badge of courage. Her bald head proudly announced to the world she was my miracle child. It was strange kissing a head of hair or being out in the "real world" with all those hairy kids! I realized I had become accustomed to seeing kids who were bald. Isn't it strange how that happens? When we first got to the hospital, every bald child made my stomach drop. The outward sign of cancer was so terrifying. It looked so unusual, so rare—something you only see on a TV commercial for St. Jude, but not in my reality, not in the world I lived in. By the time we left the hospital, when I would see children with hair, they were the ones who looked weird! Where did all that hair come from? It's amazing how your perspective changes over time. It took a while to see kids with hair and not view them as the strange ones.

YOUR MiRACLE KiD
I Told My Kid She Was a Miracle Kid, Then I Had to Prove It

From the moment Emily was diagnosed until about two weeks later it was as if I were having an out-of-body experience. I felt as if I were levitating exactly 2 inches above my body. I would look at my hand, see it was there, but feel as if it were no longer attached to me. I would stare at in wonder. I was in shock. Maybe you can relate.

A few days later, I found myself sitting at my parent conference across from the doctors ready to go over Emily's treatment plan, levitating. I distinctly remember wondering if they could tell I was floating 2 inches above where I sat. They seemed to react normally to me, so I assumed not. They began.

"So, based on Emily's lung X-rays, we are actually really surprised she was still breathing when you got here. Had you not come to the hospital and she had gone to bed that night she probably would have suffocated in her sleep. She has very advanced cancer. It has metastasized through her lungs, and we are sorry we have to tell you this, but you should know your daughter's cancer has one of the lower survival rates." I squirmed.

"It's not like leukemia with a 90% survival rate," they continued, as if somehow finding out your kid had leukemia would be cause for celebration. Since I lost a best friend in high school to leukemia, I immediately dismissed them for crazies.

Nervously I asked, "What's her cure rate?" I had to know. I prepared myself for the worst. 10 percent? 4 percent? Maybe just 1 percent? I mean I didn't know any kids who lived through cancer. "Well," they continued, "She is high risk Stage IV."

"But what is her percentage???" I pressed on. They looked at each other and then back at me, "Forty percent," they answered. I immediately realized I must have misheard. 40 was a double-digit number.

"Forty?" I reiterated, "Like 4-0?" Yes, they nodded sadly. I started to get excited! This was good news!

> **"** If you don't believe in miracles, perhaps you forgot you are one.
>
> Unknown **"**

I never told anyone what stage Emily's cancer was, yet it was one of the first questions people would ask me. At the time only my mother and sister knew. It actually was not until years later, after Emily had been transferred to the Survivor's Clinic that I would actually use the words "high risk Stage IV." When people would ask, I would simply say, "Oh I don't know; it's different in children's cancer." That seemed to satisfy their curiosity. I did this for my sake as much as for hers. I didn't want people to hear "Stage IV" and immediately equate that with a death sentence. I didn't want to see the, "there is no hope" look on their faces. And I definitely didn't want that hopeless energy transferred to my child or to her room. Remember, even if I had been told she only had a 1% survival rate, I still would have claimed her to be the 1% who survived! There is always the Miracle Kid. The kid doctors talk about, and that science can't explain. The ones who beat the odds. I wasn't going to let some protocol label of Stage IV determine my child's destiny.

"So like, almost 50! Like 50 percent!?" I exclaimed.

"Let me get this straight; Emily has the same survival rate for living through cancer as she does of getting divorced?" They looked at me oddly. "With a 50 percent success rate, people get married every day!" I continued. "Those are great odds! What a relief! Okay what's the next step to kick this tumor's butt?" I felt like I had won the lottery, and I remember the doctors looking at me completely confused.

The next day the hospital sent her pediatrician to "have a talk with me" because clearly I didn't understand the gravity of the situation. I explained that if the doctors were surprised that she was still breathing in the ER based on her X-rays, then I reasoned it was because God didn't plan on her dying, and they might know their science, but I knew it was a sign from God.

Once admitted, those few days are all still a blur, so maybe I did misunderstand, but whatever the case, in my mind I decided she was going to be a Miracle Baby, and now it was time to tell her about her Miracle Baby status.

The medical team prepared to go with me to tell Emily she had cancer. I didn't want to. I didn't want her to hear "cancer." What I didn't realize was the word "cancer" to a 3-year-old didn't carry the same heaviness and fear to her as it did to me. You could have said the flu, strep throat, or appendicitis, and they all meant the same thing. In retrospect, the staff must have thought I was nuts to think we were going to do 18 months of treatment (mostly inpatient), without her knowing she had cancer. I often wonder if they drew straws to see who was going to talk sense into the crazy mom in room 703.

Depending on your child's age, you and the medical team can decide exactly how much information you want to share with your child. At 3, Emily didn't need to know cancer can kill you. All she needed to know was that she had cancer. For many children, they already had been back and forth to doctors or had been feeling sick long before they got their cancer diagnosis. In Emily's case, she knew that for months she kept getting belly pain that caused her to curl up in my bed and cry. She knew we had seen the doctor multiple times. And now, she knew why: she had cancer.

If your hospital has a Child Life staff, they can be a huge resource in explaining what cancer means to your child. Since each cancer is somewhat different in how it represents itself (blood cancer, tumors, bone cancer, lymphoma, etc.) explaining it will vary

"Child Life specialists are pediatric health care professionals who work with children and families in hospitals and other settings to help them cope with the challenges of hospitalization, illness, and disability. ... They also provide information, support, and guidance to parents, siblings, and other family members"

GOOGLE.COM

from child to child. The easiest way we found to explain it was that all cells have a job, and when baby cells become grown up cells without learning a job, we call that cancer. Then these cells gather more and more cells that don't have jobs and start to take over the body. In Emily's case, the jobless cells all had nothing to do, so they got together and made what's called a tumor. We hated her tumor. Em called her tumor "Stupid Tumor" (stupid being a bad word at that age). If your child has leukemia or lymphoma you might picture an army of cells that turns rogue!

I then told Emily she was a Miracle Baby. What is a Miracle Baby? Well, the dictionary has one definition, but I have my own.

Miriam-Webster Dictionary: An extremely outstanding (or unusual) event, thing or accomplishment.

My Definition: A kid who does even better than the doctors predict he or she will.

Everything from then on was about proving she was a Miracle Kid. There were so many reasons why her Miracle Kid status was so important that it's hard to even begin to explain.

#1 i don't like the term "cancer kid."

The words we choose to use are powerful. We literally create our reality with the words we use. Now, this may or may not be a new realization to you! Some of us grow up in families where our parents taught us to be mindful of our words. They understood the Law of Attraction and how what we speak out into the world manifests in our life. You may have heard sayings like:

- Whatever you believe about yourself on the inside is what you will manifest on the outside. *John Assaraf*
- What you think about you bring about. *Bob Proctor*
- Never underestimate the power of the spoken word. *Kamari aka Lyrikal*
- What you're thinking is what you're becoming. *Muhammad Ali*
- What you think you become, what you feel you attract, what you imagine you create. *Buddha*
- Words kill, words give life, they are either poison or fruit. *Proverbs 18:21*
- As you think so shall you become. *Bruce Lee*
- Be careful what you think because your thoughts run your life. *Proverbs 4:23*
- I was struck by the power that the spoken word has had into determining who I am. *speakthemovie.com*
- The difference between the right word and the almost right word is the different between lightning and the lightning bug. *Mark Twain*

Or, the power of your words might be an entirely new concept to you! Maybe you've never experienced the power of your words! So here's your crash course: **"The Law of Attraction states that whatever you focus on, think about, read about, and talk about intensely, you are going to attract more of into your life."** *Jack Canfield.* I wanted my kid to be the statistic of the one who lived. So I chose to THINK about and TALK about her being a Miracle Baby! (Now that she's older she reminds me she isn't a Miracle Baby anymore, she's a Miracle Kid.) The term Cancer Kid labeled her as something I didn't want. I didn't want her to have cancer, to continue to have cancer, or to grow more cancer. To call her a Cancer Kid felt like I was covering her in a blanket of blackness and death. I wanted to cover her in light, love, and life. A Miracle.

#2 it waS fOR Me.

"Now, while she thinks she is a Miracle Baby and tells everyone, I admit I have claimed her to be one more for my sake than hers. **I need her to be a Miracle Baby.** I need her to be stronger than her cancer. I need her to kick cancer's butt. For me. Not for her. Because very openly, I have no idea what I would do without her." Yup, truth be told it was pretty selfish reasons I called her a Miracle Baby. I

was too scared not to. I decided early on to brainwash her. That SHE IS a Miracle Kid. That she WILL kick her tumor's butt. That she will WIN.

#3 MiRacle KidS KiCK CanceR'S Butt

We gave her cancer a life of its own right from the beginning. In Em's case, it was her against Stupid Tumor. If your child has a blood cancer, you simply change the language to fit your situation. For example, your child might have Stupid Cells that all swim around in their blood while white blood cells find and drown them. Or Lame Lymphomas or Bratty Bone Cancers or whatever name empowers your child and makes them feel good to call his or her cancer. Another part of giving cancer its own personality is I also wanted her to be mentally and physically separated from her cancer. She didn't "have" cancer; it wasn't part of her. Cancer was an intruder, an invader in her body, and her body was going to kick it out. We would say that Stupid Tumor didn't know she was a Miracle Kid! He just thought she was a regular kid who he could make sick, but he was wrong. We would tease Stupid Tumor and say, "You've messed with the wrroooong kid!" (Usually spoken in the general direction of her stomach where her tumor was hiding). Emily being a Miracle Kid permeated into every part of her treatment. Picture your kid like a Superhero – strong, daring, courageous, and ready to fight an evil villain (cancer). A Miracle Kid is way more fun, upbeat, and life giving than a Cancer Kid, don't you think?

Em had a personal vendetta against Stupid Tumor. She talked to it and teased it. She told it she was going to kill it. She told me one night she wanted me to take a water gun, shoot it up to heaven, make God come down, cut open her belly, take out her tumor, and throw it out the window. Sounded like a good plan to me.

Just like all Superheros, Miracle Kids fight off evil villains—theirs is just called cancer. Like all Superheroes, Miracle Kids have their own arsenal of weapons at their disposal to help declare victory. Their weapons include chemo, medicine, transfusions, broviacs, ports, face masks, and more. There will also be more chances to use your Yes and Making Cancer Fun training. YES cancer is trying to win AND you have weapons to fight back. Victory will be yours!

Here's a Peek into the World of My Miracle Kid and How She fought Cancer and Won.

Em had a clot. It was in her shoulder. She had to get painful leg injections twice daily. It stunk, for both of us. I would feel like an evil child abuser leading her by the hand into the bathroom to administer said evil shot while she screamed and cried. I would cry too sometimes. I explained to her that her tumor told her red blood cells to get together and have a party. The tumor was vindictive like that. He'd get the red blood cells to do things they knew they shouldn't do. So her red blood was hanging out in her shoulder and having a block party and blocking up traffic. The other red blood can't get through. Her leg med was like the police. The medicine would go up into her shoulder and tell the red blood, "Hey break it up! Break it up!" (Which, of course, is said in a tough NYC cop voice.) This made sense to Em. She would tell her shoulder, "Break it up!"

We would talk about chemo. Chemo was our friend. It would go into her body and do karate on her tumor. I would then act out crazy karate poses, air kicks, and punches around the hospital room. This is, of course, what her chemo did to the tumor. The tumor was scared of chemo. We do Karate Fox Chemo. Aunt Laura brought us stickers that have animals doing karate, which we would stick to her chemo tubes and all over her belly. I would put my mouth close to her belly and say, "Hey tumor! We're doing chemo! What's that? Oh you're scared? Run home to your mommy and cry tumor...you're getting your butt kicked today!" Then I would turn my ear to her belly and say, "Em do you hear that? Your tumor is crying and screaming!" She loved to do anything to make Stupid Tumor cry.

Emily had a Broviac—two implanted IV lines in her chest. (Broviacs are one of the special weapons Miracle Kids have so they can beat cancer.) One line had a red tip, and one had a white. We called them "Champions" because they helped deliver champion fighting chemo. They would often argue with each other over who would get flushed first, or who would get to give the lab draw, or who would get hooked up to chemo. "Pick me! Pick me!" you could often hear them shouting. Of course Emily was in charge, so she always had the final say. Her champions were her friends, but they could be very silly and dramatic at times.

Em needed an X-ray almost every day for two months: one every morning and sometimes during the day. I would tell her she took such great pictures that they needed more. (After all, Miracle Kids are rare. Doctors are intrigued by them.) Sometimes she would stick out her tongue, and we would laugh wondering what the doctors would say when they saw her tongue sticking out in her in pictures!

Emily also needed breathing treatments four times a day for three months. I'll never forget the first time the Respiratory Therapist (RT) came into the room. He wanted to put an oxygen mask over Em's mouth and have her breathe into it against the air to get her lungs to expand. She screamed and screamed. Some big plastic mask over your face would be scary, don't you think?

I asked the therapist, "What do you do if they won't stop screaming?" You know what he told me? "We let them scream...it helps open their lungs anyway."

Uh what?!?!

There was no way an RT was coming four times a day to make my kid scream in fear. That was not going to fly. We needed to change our strategy, fast. The next time I asked for a breathing mask for myself. I told Em I was a better breather and I could breathe faster than she could. I dared her to race me. It took a bit of reverse psychology, until she realized how fun it was to beat mom. Miracle Kids always win after all.

Many times we adjusted the "game" based on the treatment. It could be a race to see who could breathe faster into the plastic or maybe see who could blow harder into the plastic. Miracle Kids breathe the strongest. We could adjust it, but it was always a race. My piece, of course, was not hooked up to a machine or to the oxygen the way hers was. Mine was just an empty plastic piece, so this was really about harnessing the imagination of a child! I would always try to "win," and she would always win instead. I will be soooo dramatic blowing as hard as I could, and somehow Emily always won. She thought it was hysterical to always beat her mom at her breathing treatments. Imagine how fun it is to a child to see mom try as hard as she can, breathing hard and falling

backwards onto the bed because she is so out of breath! Giggles everywhere!

What we were racing for I'm still not sure, except I would count to fifteen and then pretend I was totally out of breath. I would make a big deal to the RT that Em always beat me and that she was a show-off. In the end, Em would actually hold the mask to her face and breathe herself, which all the RT people told me they had never seen a 3-year-old do. I reminded them they had never seen my Miracle Kid.

Em lived on the "Bear Floor." At our hospital each floor had an animal. The oncology floor was the "Bear Floor." Oh, how many days and months we spent on the "Bear Floor." Often, when Emily and I would be on the elevator together and people would exit off onto other floors, we would look knowingly at each other and say, "They're not going to the Bear Floor!" I mean,

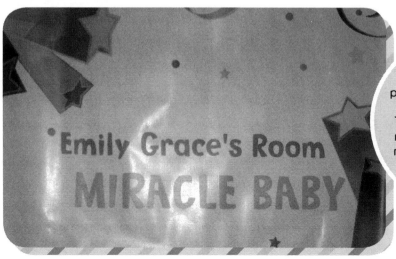

Emily Grace's Room
MIRACLE BABY

I had this poster printed shortly after her diagnosis. Truth be told, this was more for me to remind myself that she was my Miracle Baby.

we knew that only the coolest people, the best of the best, the strongest and bravest got to go to the bear floor! Only Miracle Kids are allowed on the "Bear Floor." These little silly's make day-to-day hospital life a little more bear-able, hehehe.

Miracle Kids go "cruising." This is what we called it anytime they had to transport Em through the hospital to have a scan or X-ray done. Going to new rooms was no longer scary, it became fun. I would sit in the bed with her, and we would "cruise." (I don't think the parents were supposed to sit on the bed, but no one ever said anything). Miracle Kids also need sidekicks. (Don't all superheroes?) Our sidekicks just happened to be an array of stuffed animals. We would make a big production of which stuffed animals got the "privilege" of going cruising with us. Which ones had gotten to cruise before? Which ones would behave the best? Pup once got sent home because he always wanted to go roller skating down those long, shiny, perfect skating halls. He also got himself a girlfriend named Pickles. She was the stuffed dog the CAT scanner guy gave Em one time because everyone thought she was fun. She named the new dog Pickles. Pup fell for Pickles fast and the

whole romance was enacted out on the "cruise" back to our room. Moose the hand puppet was well known for cruising because he High-Fived everyone in the halls. He did this whether they wanted to High-Five back or not. Most people loved to play along except for one doctor who literally backed away from me in the elevator. (Seriously? You work in a children's hospital!) Frog would slide down the hall handrails and go "Weeee!" Piggy would climb up and down the elevator walls. One day Parasol the Pony slid all over the strange, scary, space-age scanning machine that freaked Em out and then went on its "water slide" to show her how it wasn't scary at all. Miracle Kids have the most fun.

Emily was very interested in what was going to happen to Stupid Tumor after he was taken out of her. I explained that he went to Pathology. "What happens in Pathology?" she wanted to know. I told her this is where all the tumors went. I explained part of the problem with tumors is no one knows how her tumor got into her and doctors don't know how tumors get into other kids either. Because she was a Miracle Kid and she had kicked her tumor out, he was now going to get taken to Pathology where he was

tHe SunSHine Kid

If your child has siblings it can be hard to make sure they don't feel left out. After all, Miracle Kid status could be perceived as something to be jealous of. The Miracle Kid is suddenly getting all of mom's and dad's time and attention. Fortunately, siblings have their own special Superhero status. They are Sunshine Kids. Their super power is that they bring sunshine to everyone they meet. When they visit their Miracle Kid sibling....sunshine! When their parents are feeling sad about cancer....sunshine! The Miracle Kid needs a Sunshine Kid(s) to keep them going. Just like Superman gets his powers from the energy of the yellow star, Miracle Kids get stronger when they are around Sunshine Kids. Their Sunshine Kid status gives you an opportunity to remind your child how important he or she still is. You can point out all the wonderful things they do to bring sunshine into the world. For example their "contagious laugh" (pun intended), how helpful they are around the house, how patient they are during doctor's visits, or how loving they are to the Miracle Kid. You can even make it fun by giving your Sunshine Kid a special sun-shaped wand, flashlight, or yellow glow stick to bring sun to the Miracle Kid!

going to get poked, chopped, cut up, and even have fire put on him. (OK, I have no clue what happens in pathology, but these were all the things I wanted to see happen to him!) Her little eyes would light up at this idea. She loved to picture tumor being tortured every day and every night forever. (Very brimstone and fire like we were.)

I also explained that Tumor had no friends because the other tumors were so mad at him. After all, he had accidentally picked a Miracle Kid to mess with and that Miracle Kid had kicked his butt all the way to Pathology. Now scientists and doctors were going to figure out how tumors got into kids by studying her tumor so they would actually be able to stop other tumors from getting into other kids! Of course all the other tumors were really mad at Stupid Tumor because he was ruining it for all of them. He had messed with the wrong kid. How stupid was he? We would mimic how the other tumors were making fun of Stupid Tumor. "You stupid tumor, why did you mess with a Miracle Kid?" or "You're not our friend, and we don't like you!" Then we would also act out Stupid Tumor crying and wailing, "No stop! Don't poke at me! Ouch!!!" Em would laugh and laugh.

We would often talk about how great it was that Tumor was in Pathology, and we would try to think of all the horrible things that might be happening to him that day. How many pokes he got, how many chops he got. Emily loved the idea of torturing Stupid Tumor on a regular basis and especially that Stupid Tumor had no friends anymore because everyone was mad at him for messing with a Miracle Kid. Every now and then when Emily had to do something that was really hard, like a leg poke or scary procedure, we would stop, put our hand to our ears and say, "Do you hear that?" She would grin at me, and I would grin at her. We would say it was Stupid Tumor screaming, "No!

Don't do it! Don't Do it!" Then when she would do whatever she needed to do he would cry louder "NO!!!!" It really was Em versus Stupid Tumor.

At one point Em didn't want to eat, because every time she would eat she would throw up. She had a feeding tube in, and we couldn't get the feeding tube out until she started eating again on her own. I would put food in front of her, and she would just look at it. I'd say to her, "Emily, Stupid Tumor doesn't want you to eat this. He wants you to stay sick. He wants you to stay weak." She would look at me, narrow her eyes and take a bite. There was no way she was going to let him win. I believe it was Emily's fighting spirit, her strong will, and her determination that helped her not give up.

We recently took an online personality test. The type where you look at pictures and choose what you see or what color stands out. I came back with kindness as my dominate trait. Emily's? Courage. Yup, courage. Her courage helped her not want to throw in the towel or say, "I can't do it, and it's too hard." I believe every child can be courageous if they are empowered by those around them. I doubt she understood that at 3 and 4 years old that she set the expectation for the rest of her life. There's nothing that's too hard for her to accomplish. There's nothing too difficult for her. She is a Miracle Kid after all. She kicked cancer at three. When she was scared about starting kindergarten, nervous about leaving me and going with the other new kids that would be there, I would say to her, "Emily you don't under-stand. You are already so ahead of these other kids. These kids are just learning to sit in a circle, learning to keep their hands to themselves, learning how to not pick their nose! But you? You kicked cancer's butt at 3. As you grow up and someone says to you 'Emily you can't do that!' or 'Emily that's too hard!' or 'Oh Emily no one's ever done that before!' you can look them in the eye and say 'Don't tell me what I can't do, I kicked cancer at 3!'" I pray with all my heart that she keeps that cou-rageous spirit the rest of her life. As obsta-cles come up, and as life tries to knock her down, I hope she will stand firm remem-bering that she is a Miracle Kid.

REMEMBER:

The key with the Sunshine Kid is not just to be the Miracle Kid's sidekick, but to be their OWN special Superhero that is equally important!

PEOPLE WILL ASK ABOUT YOUR MIRACLE KID.

Just like all well-known Superheroes, no one knew they were Superheroes until the had a public battle with a nemesis. As people find out about your child's Miracle Kid Status they will probably be shocked (not every-one meets a Miracle Kid every day you know) and they will be curious and ask questions. It is a personal decision how much your family wants to share with others. People will ask your child's cancer stage. Determine ahead of time how you (and your spouse/family) will answer that question.

CONSIDER:

How will someone else's reaction affect you? Will it trigger fear in you? Will it trigger fear in your child? Will someone's reaction open up more questions for your child that you might not be ready to answer?

Just Because someone asks a question, it doesn't mean you have to answer it.

Fun Factor

What type of cancer does your child have?

_____

If you had to give it a personality, what would it be like?

_____

_____

_____

Have your child come up with a name for his/her cancer (the Villain):

_____

What would it look like?

Fun Factor

What are some of the Weapons your Miracle Kid has to fight cancer?

- ○ Chemotherapy (Karate Fox Chemo!)
- ○ A Broviac or Port
- ○ Oxygen Mask/Tube
- ○ An IV Pole
- ○ A wide variety of superhero pills and liquids (medicine)
- ○ Feeding Tubes (to administer superhero food)
- ○ TPN (advanced Superhero food)
- ○ A flying Hospital Bed that moves up and down and cruises the halls
- ○ A Hospital Room—Most Superheroes have a "secret base"
- ✓ _____
- ✓ _____
- ✓ _____

Doctors are fascinated with Miracle Kids. They are constantly studying them. What are some things Miracle Kids do that "normal" kids don't get to do?

- ○ Radiation
- ○ X-Ray
- ○ GAT/PET Scan
- ○ Ultrasound
- ○ MRI
- ○ Biopsy
- ○ Surgery
- ✓ _____
- ✓ _____
- ✓ _____

What do Miracle Kids wear?

- ○ Superhero hospital gown
- ○ Superhero face masks to protect them from germs (cancer villain's allies)
- ○ Superhero slippers
- ○ Miracle Kids are usually bald, too! It's a sign of their Superhero status.
- ✓ _____
- ✓ _____
- ✓ _____
- ✓ _____

Fun Factor

Does your Miracle Kid have any Sunshine Kids in his or her life?
If yes, what are their unique personality qualities that can contribute to helping the Miracle Kid?

* Are they musical? Do they sing or play an instrument? Maybe they can come up with their own Miracle Kid and the Sunshine Band!

* Are they artistic? Can they make pictures, art, or crafts to decorate the Miracle Kid's room? Maybe all with a sunshine theme?

* Are they funny? Do they tell jokes to make the Miracle Kid laugh? Maybe buy them a joke book and have them pick out their favorites for a stand-up routine they will perform for the Miracle Kid.

* Are they gentle? Can they sit with the Miracle Kid and hold their hand? Share a favorite stuffed animal? Read to the Miracle Kid?

* Are they an encourager? Maybe they can get yellow sunshine pompoms, toy sunshine wands, or yellow glow sticks to cheer on the Miracle Kid and tell them, "You can do it!"

* _____
  _____
  _____
  _____
  _____

* _____
  _____
  _____
  _____
  _____

Prove it

Kids are smart. They figure things out….quickly. We, as parents, need to be quicker. Be prepared to defend your child's Miracle Kid status. Emily wasn't going to take it at face value that she was a Miracle Baby. I had to prove to her that she was. Here are some examples of my "proof."

★ Only Miracle Babies puked golden puke – even Aunt Chrissy the nurse knew this. (I assumed oncology kids puked all sorts of colors, but we never saw their puke, only Emily's.)

★ When we would arrive at the ER they would take her right into her room. She didn't need to wait in the waiting room like the other "non-miracle" babies. (By the way all oncology kids are taken right in so they don't catch germs from the waiting room.)

★ Molly, one of the nurses, did a Miracle Baby exam on her. (The exam was because Emily was going to take an anti-nausea drug they had never used on a child under 7 before.)

★ Ann, one of our nurses, said she never has seen the "Diamond Cut" before. (Fortunately Ann was quick on her feet too and caught on fast. Emily was cut across her stomach like a triangle instead of a traditional line because of the location of her tumor.)

★ At 6:30 am in the surgery waiting room we were the only ones there. We concluded they must only operate on Miracle Kids on Monday because it's "Miracle Monday." (Oh and because technically I don't think the surgery room opened before 8 but hers was such a long surgery we had to get there early.) There was a baby that showed up, so the baby must have been a Miracle Kid too, but we were certain he must have gotten the "Line" cut not the "Diamond" cut, further confirming only Miracle Babies got surgery on Mondays.

★ Miracle Babies got nose tubes…other kids had to take their meds by mouth.

★ Miracle Babies only spent one day in the PICU after surgery.

★ Emily asked, "Mom what day do I get my surgery?" I answered, "Miracle Monday Em." She looked at me seriously and said, "I bet other kids get theirs on Tuesday or Thursday."

★ Miracle Babies were on the Bear Floor. (the oncology floor) Ashley the receptionist wouldn't let other kids on it.

★ When people stared at her in the "real world" it's because she was a Miracle Baby…and then we pointed out who was staring.

★ Miracle Babies got Santa to personally visit them. (And moms who had amazing friends who also happened to be actors.)

★ Miracle Babies got visits from Dr. Ben who no longer worked on the oncology floor but still came to visit.

★ Miracle Babies got Facebook Fan Pages.

★ Miracle Babies got X-Rays every day.

A Peek Into Our World—Making Cancer Fun and Other Things that Offend People

Written March 13, 2010 at 8:38pm — 4 months into treatment

Emily looked up at me two days ago and said, "I want to call my tumor a bad word."

"What?" I asked her.

"I want to call it a damn tumor."

I, of course, said, "No, we can't do that."

She looked at me with all the exasperation a 3-year-old can muster and said, "Why not? It is a damn tumor."

Now it was hard for me to explain that while we hate the tumor and yes, it is in fact, a damn tumor we can't actually call it a damn tumor because damn is a bad word. I could see the wheels of confusion spinning in her little brain. "But why can't I call it damn tumor? I don't like it!" I agreed, after all it's a f*ckin damn tumor, I think to myself. I calmly explain using the word "damn" makes us sound trashy, and we don't want our tumor to make us trashy. I don't think she bought it.

I notice how many people are always commenting on how positive I am. I'm becoming more aware that it is a choice. Sometimes I think, "That's just me." However, when things have been hard, like last week, (Emily had been running 104.5 temps we couldn't break...and had pain in her intestines that was keeping her on a narcotic drip...and couldn't talk and stayed in bed with mucus dripping out of her blood-stained mouth...and the Doctors weren't sure if it was an infection causing the swelling of her intestines or if possibly just possibly the chemo had destroyed the integrity of her intestines or maybe her immune system was turning on itself and attacking her intestines.) Yeah, I was stressed and I was scared, and I thought, "Did we come this far for nothing? Has she been this strong for nothing?" I wanted to slip into the land of fear...and let it overtake me and paralyze me. And then I made the choice. "NO! She will be Ok." I reminded myself she has come this far. She is strong, she is a fighter and this is just part of her fight.

We talk about her 5-year-old birthday. (She wants a "pink water kitty:" a cat that can play in the pool with her and obviously, is pink. When I explain I have never seen a pink cat, she doesn't hesitate to point out Strawberry Shortcake has a pink kitty, and so she can have one too.)

We talk about her 6-year-old birthday...we want the whole family to take a Disney Cruise together to celebrate her 2-year anniversary for her bone marrow transplant. (That's when the doctors have said I can breathe again...never normal breathing of course, but at least full breaths.)

We talk about her starting school...how when other kids are told they "can't" in life they will think they can't. When someone tells Emily she "can't" she will look at her courage beads and say, "YES I CAN!"

We talk about her learning to drive and how scared I'll be and how I'll wish we were back on the "Bear Floor" because that was less scary!

We talk about her prom, going to college, getting married, and what a great mom she'll be.

We talk in detail. Filling her subconscious with expectations it WILL fulfill.

Tonight she is lying next to me as I type this. Hooked into her IV pole, her little arm is twisted up and around my bicep while she listens to Taylor Swift (her favorite) with her eyes closed. She had tried singing earlier but her throat is still too swollen. She had looked up at me and asked, "Mommy when we go to Brent's place (where she'll stay after we discharge next from the hospital) will I be able to talk normal again?"

"Yes, Em you will, I promise," I had said "It hurts to sing, huh?" I asked and she nodded.

I rub lotion on her feet, her legs, her arms, her hands, her back, and her bald head. I go to rub lotion on her scars. The two deep ones on her right side. One where a chest tube stayed implanted into her for more than two months. The other where a second chest tube stayed for over a month. The two month one is deep and wide. It was put into her in the ER when she was first admitted. It was a, "stick this in to get that fluid out, she should be dead already, who cares what it looks like" scar, and the now "famous" "Diamond Cut" the 8-inch cut across her abdomen where they took her tumor out.

She pushes my hand away. "No," she says.

"Em, let me put lotion on those scars because it will help them heal."

"No," she says. "I want them."

"Why do you want them?"" I ask giving her a look of exasperation.

She snuggles up under her hospital sheet. "Because they'll remind me how brave I am"

She might just be the bravest, strongest person I've ever met. I look at her in awe, keenly aware I'm looking at a living, breathing, miracle.

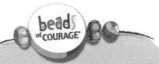

"Beads of Courage helps more than 60,000 children in eight countries, record, tell, and own their stories using colorful beads as meaningful symbols of courage and hope along their treatment journey."

www.beadsofcourage.org

PARTY PLANNING 101
The Only Party Not to Throw
Is a Pity Party

One of my core Making Cancer Fun ideas is to turn everything into a party. In first grade when Emily completed her two-year off-treatment follow-up visit for a full two days at the hospital, she went back to school and told her classmates and her teacher that the reason she had been gone was because she was at a party with her mom. That is how my daughter, at 6 years old, viewed her follow-up treatments. Everything was a party.

Having parties will serve lots of purposes. Parties give you something to look forward to, a reason to have fun, and sometimes they even help explain what is going on medically. I honestly thought everyone was throwing parties and trying to have fun all the time! Now get ready, if you aren't already, you're about to become an A+ party planner!

OUR fiRST BiG PARTY: OH NO the BiG 5-0!

Our first big party came on day 50. We had been at the hospital 50 days straight. I went to the party store, found 50th birthday celebration supplies and improvised. Streamers that I could hang from the top of the ceiling that said "50," a huge basket of purple beaded necklaces to hand out to all of the staff, and even a button that lit up and said, "Oh no, the big 5-0." I found a big matching necklace that also said, "Oh no, the big 5-0" for Emily to wear. We got party plates. We got napkins. We got cups. We threw a party right there in the hospital room! Now, coincidentally, this was also the day they decided to harvest her stem cells for her bone marrow transplant.

Emily's cancer was never actually in her blood. That was one of the reasons why it was so difficult to get her diagnosed early on, because her blood work kept coming back normal. The way it worked with Emily's neuroblastoma was the hospital could harvest her body's own stem cells, freeze them, and wait until her transplant to then transplant her own stem cells back into her own body. So that's what we did.

> *Laughter is an instant vacation.*
>
> *Milton Berle*

the truth about bone marrow transplants

So many families sit, wait, hope, and worry as to whether or not they'll have a donor. Scared can't begin to describe the emotions these parents must feel. Because Emily's cancer never was in her blood, we didn't have that fear. We knew she could be her own donor. However, I met so many families that didn't have that luxury. That's why I'm such an advocate of joining the bone marrow transplant registry www.bethematch.org. It's simple. You literally get your mouth wiped with a Q-tip and get on the bone marrow transplant list. You can save the life of a person who is waiting desperately for your bone marrow. It is not a big procedure or a painful process. I sat there and watched Emily have her stem cells taken out of her arm, just like an IV.

What most people don't realize is that in order to get a bone marrow transplant, you need to be cancer-free. That means that your chemo has to be successful. Often what happens is a child can't get to a place where they're cancer-free in order to have their transplant. One of the families I fell most in love with lost their beautiful son, Zack, after a second relapse of leukemia, simply because every time he got close enough to get ready for his transplant, his body still showed he had an infection or that there were still active cancer cells. I watched this family struggle with having a perfect ten match donor, but he never actually got to transplant. Zack is now a beautiful angel, who watches over us from heaven.

Another reason why people can't get through a bone marrow transplant is they simply don't have a donor who matches. The closer the match, the larger success rate. The lower the match, the higher the chances of the body rejecting it with graft-versus-host disease. Your donor could be from anyone, anywhere. A lot of times family members simply don't match, or they don't match up enough, and the risk of the transplant is too great. So, if nothing else, put this book down and go get on the bone marrow transplant registry. Your little swab of spit could literally save somebody's life. Someone who right now is counting the days, because once that person is cancer-free, they will have only so many days before getting transplant. If the cancer starts to come back, that person might not be eligible for the transplant, and at that point, there may be no other options to cure the cancer. You could be the one person who is the only match.

The nurses brought in this huge machine that took up half the room. Emily had to sit there all day with a nurse, who monitored it. They hooked up her broviac (IV lines), and I watched as they spun her cells out of her body through the machine, taking out her stem cells and putting her blood back into her. They had to collect so many cells per hour. At the halfway mark, she was above what she needed. My little Miracle Baby, her stem cells were excited and ready. We talked about how her stem cells were going to "Boot Camp" (more on Boot Camp later!). They were going to go learn how to kick cancer's butt, and they were coming out of her body. They were going to learn how to help her kick Stupid Tumor out of her for good. Because we were having such a big party, and we had lots of nurses who didn't normally treat us, they definitely thought our room was a little wacky. We gave everyone party beads to wear for the day. We asked everyone coming by to sign the fifty-day party poster hanging on her door. We decorated her room with lots of streamers. "Oh no, the big 5-0," became the fun saying of the day. Em loved handing out party favors, shaking her booty, and dancing in bed a lot. (The best she could "dance" hooked up to so many wires!) The real question is how much fun can you have harvesting stem cells?

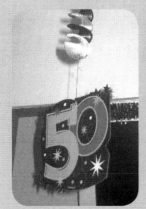
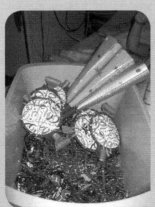
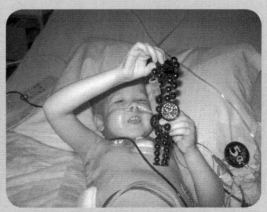

Party favors in a puke bucket.

Cancer Will Become a Blur and Parties Help Our Brains Remember the Good Stuff

When you're going through childhood cancer it's hard to think that at some point cancer will be a memory. It feels like forever. Believe it or not, it's hard sometimes to remember all the silly things we did during Emily's treatment. The good thing about getting through cancer is that it does start to become a blur. As with all memories, it's only the really "big" things that stick out in our minds. So the goal with parties is that the FUN will be the "big" thing our kids remember most.

Having parties for hitting bench marks is easy. We did two parties based on time milestones—the 50 day party you just read about and a 75-day party. You can choose a number of days for hospital stays, a number of chemos completed, anniversary days (1-year since diagnosis, 1-year since first chemo, etc.) or hitting a certain part of treatment (for example if you know your roadmap is an 18-month treatment plan you can celebrate at the 6-month, 12-month, and 18-month mark!) Let's break down the 75-day party so can see how simple planning the perfect party can be!

Wearing a "mommy hug" (my tank top) at the 75-day party.

Choose a Fun Theme: We chose "High-Five the 75," and we started hi-fiving everyone who came in during the day.

Make a Party Pack: Something as easy as swapping out traditional hospital plates, napkins, and cups with party plates, napkins, and cups can make a kid ready to party! For our 75-day party I couldn't find themed 75-day supplies, so I just used celebration ones that were blue with streamers on them!

Decorate: Often you can find birthday decorations to use for benchmark parties. 1-year old birthday decorations for anniversary parties, 6-year old decorations for 6-month parties, 3-year old decorations for third chemo treatment parties, etc. Or the dollar store always has generic (and cheap!) decorations. Streamers are easy to hang, balloons (ask the hospital first what they allow), or grab some paper, paints, and markers and make your own. (It serves two purposes: making decorations and keeping boredom at bay!) For the 75-day party, since I couldn't find 75-themed decorations, I just hung colored streamers!

Get a Poster for Friends, Family, and Staff to Sign: We didn't do this for every party, but for our big ones we did. For the 75-day party I found a 75th birthday poster I hung on her door. Other times I just used a huge poster board and wrote the party theme in marker across the top. Again, you could decorate your poster with stickers and markers with your child and then hang it up! Ask staff members to write a note of encouragement to your child. Most are happy to! They love that you are doing your part to keep the patient happy—a happy child usually equals a cooperative child! These words of encouragement also build your child's spirit when he or she reads how "strong," "courageous," and "brave," the staff thinks he or she is!

Hand Out Party Favors: Keep it simple and keep it cheap! (The motto for all of my parties!) Party stores usually have lots of silly children's party favors to hand out! For the 75-day party I think we did Hershey kisses. Individually wrapped mints, mini M&M's, buttons, party beads, plastic bracelets, Ring Pops, etc. all work. Sometimes our favors matched our themes, and sometimes they were just candy. (Don't worry the staff loves candy!)

Choose a Song:

We chose the song "Celebration" by Kool and the Gang as our theme song for the day. I have two videos from that day—one of Em laying in bed, passed out from all her steroids and medication in my tank top that barely fit her because she wanted a mommy "hug" around her and an earlier video of her and her little bald head, sitting on a bench with her food in front of her and the party plate, singing and fist pumping like she was from Jersey to "Celebration." Which do you think I remember taking? We sang, "There's a party going on in here. A celebration to last throughout the year. Bring your good times and your laughter too. We're gonna celebrate a party with you. Come on now." I danced like crazy around the room, which of course made Emily dissolve into a bundle of laughter.

> We were planning on having an 80 or 100-day party, but we finally checked out on day 78, never quite making it to the eightieth day. Yes that's right, from the time we checked into the emergency room two days before Thanksgiving, not knowing what was wrong, it was seventy-eight days later before we finally checked out of the hospital. It was a momentous day of actually going home for the first time. Sadly, we were only home for a few days before Emily ran a fever and we were right back in the hospital.

Parties can Help explain Stuff too

In addition to celebrating, I used Emily's parties to explain what was happening to her medically. Below are a few parties that cancer kids might need to throw! My goal is to give you a peek into how my brain worked—my YES, and, + a Party!

> When we experience victory in the face of obstacles I believe it gives us glimpses into God's divine hand in our lives.

Have you ever Stomped on a tumor?

Not every child who has cancer will need surgery or have a tumor. But if your kid is a "tumor" Cancer Kid, be ready to give that tumor a life of its own. YES, Emily had a tumor AND he was his own person, so we were going to kick his butt and throw a party! Emily named her tumor "Stupid Tumor," and we hated him (I still do). When Emily had to do things she didn't want to do we would talk about how "Stupid Tumor" was teasing and taunting her and how she had to be stronger than him and kick his butt! Here's how we threw a Tumor Stomping party! (It's still my favorite party!)

I had given her surgeon my camera before the surgery and asked her if she would take a couple of pictures of Stupid Tumor. She was happy to oblige and later gave us an assortment of disgusting bloody pictures. (Have you ever seen someone's insides before?) I didn't expect, when I got the camera back, I would be looking at stuff that was basically unrecognizable. Only the small view of a little belly button made me realize it was Emily's stomach, cut open, looking like a raw piece of meat. It was disgusting and made me want to vomit. Gross! Emily loved it!

I was shocked at how small Stupid Tumor was and how something so tiny could threaten one person's life so much. Like the power of one single bullet. It was a disgustingm bloody piece of mass, and I have never hated anything that looked so gross in all my life.

I brought the pictures of Stupid Tumor over to my local copy store. I asked them to blow one of them up into a huge poster. I'm sure those employees must have secretly questioned my sanity. I also asked them to make lots of color copies of it too! First, I hung the poster of the tumor on her wall. Then I took the 8x10 pictures of her tumor and scattered them around the floor. I had picked up in a dollar bin cute little banana slippers for Emily to wear as her special "tumor stomping" slippers to "stomp" her tumor with. We also had these long plastic shooters that the staff used to help children with their breathing exercises. You would put a marshmallow in it and blow as hard as you could to shoot the marshmallow across the room. It was just one of the many games that the hospital staff would use with the kids to help them expand their lungs and breathe. We decided that the marshmallow shooters had a much better purpose, shooting tumors. We bought cupcakes and had friends come to visit. We were ready.

I helped Emily slip on her banana slippers. We starting blaring Miley Cyrus' "Party in the USA," and holding onto her IV pole, she slowly stomped her way around the room smashing each tumor picture with her tiny feet. Then she sat on the floor and physically ripped up all the pictures into tiny pieces while we all yelled at the tumor and told it how much we hated him. She then sat on her bed and began to shoot the large poster of her tumor with marshmallows and telling Stupid Tumor to, "Take that!" All the nurses came in, and they took turns

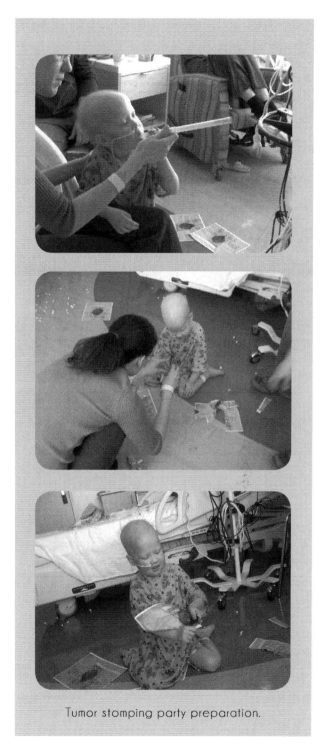

Tumor stomping party preparation.

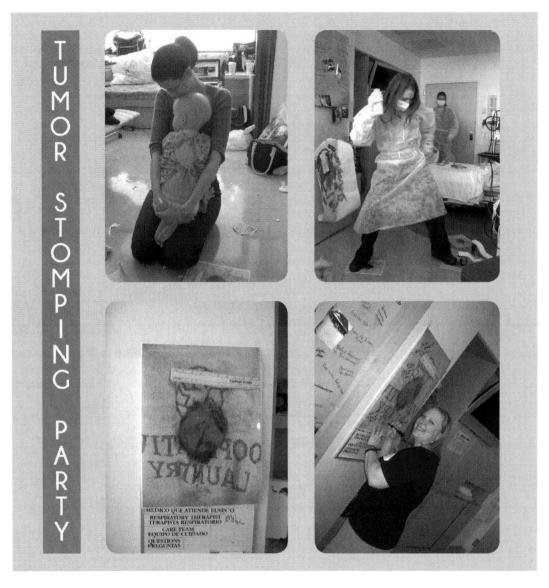

TUMOR STOMPING PARTY

stomping on the tumor pictures and writing her congratulations on her tumor poster. (Which also involved telling the tumor it could take a hike!) I hope she values that poster one day when she's older. All the signatures, all those people cheering her on, making fun of tumor, telling him he was too weak for a Miracle Kid, and then celebrating with cupcakes. I don't know that she really remembers her surgery. And she doesn't remember the eight hours she was under anesthesia, but she definitely remembers the fun she had at her tumor stomping party!

Bone Marrow Parties are actually Boot Camp for Stem Cells

Some children will have to face going through a bone marrow transplant. Unlike other theme parties that can be based solely on easily available (and cheap) decorations, this theme party can be an extension of how to explain to your child what is going on medically.

If your child uses his or her own stem cells (the way Emily did) you'll actually start talking about Boot Camp that day. If your child uses donor stem cells then you could approach it a few ways. First, let me explain how Boot Camp works.

To explain why Emily needed to have her stem cells taken out, I told her that her cells were going off to Boot Camp, where they were going to learn how to kick cancer's butt. I explained to her that when we took tumor out of her all of her cancer was gone. (I really wanted her to mentally be in a place where once the tumor was gone, it wasn't coming back and there wouldn't be any fear of it returning. Obviously, at the innocent age of 4, all she knew was what I choose to tell her.) I told her that chemo had killed the cancer, the tumor had come out and it wasn't in her anymore. But, we were still afraid that there might

be some cells in her body that would be "traitor cells." Now, of course, a 4-year old doesn't know what a traitor is, so I explained a traitor is somebody who maybe is still friends with tumor. We didn't want anybody in her body who would still be friends with Stupid Tumor! So her stem cells were going to Boot Camp to learn how to look for traitors and to help kick cancer's butt.

On her bone marrow transplant (BMT) day her cells would be coming back from Boot Camp all prepared to help by going into her body and searching around to find out if there were any traitors left. If they did indeed find a traitor, of course, they would kick its butt! I described how her stem cells would take their tanks and their guns and they would be ready to shoot and knock down any cell that might be a traitor.

Helpful Hint

If you use donor cells you could explain early on that you have special "Miracle Stem Cells" waiting for their transplant day. This could be used as "proof" of Miracle Kid status. Or if you are getting stem cells from a family member you could explain their sisters/brothers/cousin's stem cells decided they wanted to join in on the fight so they "enlisted" (just like they do in the Army) meaning they signed up to join in fighting cancer. Of course, just like Army soldiers who don't sign up and head right to war, they have to go through Boot Camp first to learn to fight. So the Stem Cells have gone to boot camp and are coming back to go to war on cancer. You could even use this explanation as a positive mental piece—your child has been hard at work to get to BMT all on his or her own, but pretty soon BMT reinforcements will be coming to help. Remember, being a cancer fun maker is like going back to being a kid yourself. When a broom was a flying stick, a pot a drum, and a cardboard box was a boat, space ship, or anything your imagination wanted it to be. Are you willing to find your inner child to make cancer fun?

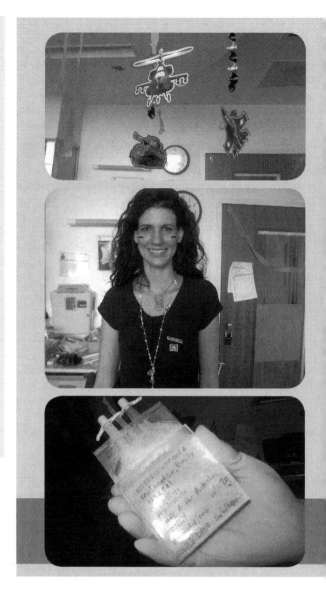

Holding a Boot Camp party is super simple because there are so many Army-themed party celebrations. We hung Army tank decorations from the ceiling. I got a big green poster for everyone to sign and decorated it with Army stickers. I bought little tags that looked like military dog tags from the party supply store so Emily and the nurses could wear them, and we gave everyone a title. There was the first lieutenant in command, the five-star general and others based on their rank. Emily of course was top dog!

In the oncology world a BMT is often called a second birthday. Until she was 9 and transferred to the Survivor's Clinic we celebrated her second birthday every year.

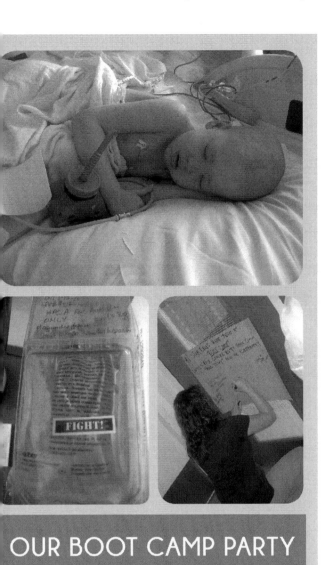

OUR BOOT CAMP PARTY

UNDERSTANDING BMT IN LAYMAN'S TERMS

Cancer cells grow and divide quickly. Chemotherapy kills these rapidly growing cancer cells. It can affect normal cells that grow fast too like the cells that make hair or blood. Chemotherapy can interfere with the body's ability to produce red blood cells, white blood cells, and platelets. Most normal cells can regenerate, but the patient may need transfusions in the meantime. Patients can experience what's called "neutropenia" meaning they have less than a 500 white blood cell count causing very low immunity. During this time the patient waits for that number to go up and up, watching as the white blood cells rebuild themselves.

Chemo is usually given with breaks between treatment cycles. The breaks give your body time to rebuild healthy new cells. When the doses of chemo and radiation needed to cure a cancer are so high that the stem cells are permanently damaged or destroyed by treatment, a bone marrow transplant is needed.

THERE ARE TWO TYPES OF TRANSPLANTS

Autologous Transplant: This is where patients can use their own stem cells to replace the bone marrow and restore its function (after those high doses of chemo and radiation were given to destroy the cancer). The stem cells are taken from the patient (either by bone marrow harvest or apheresis, which is a process of collecting peripheral blood stem cells) and frozen. Later, the stem cells are transplanted back into the patient after intensive treatment.

Allogeneic Transplant: In this case the stem cells are taken from a genetically matched donor. The closer the match (10/10 being perfect) the less chance the body will reject them.

These stem cells are what create the white blood cells, red blood cells, and platelets that our body needs. Without replacing these stems cells a patient couldn't survive. There would be no immune system left. When you transplant those stem cells back you are waiting for those new cells to graft into the body and to start to produce new white blood cells.

There is not a way to predict how long this grafting process will take. You simply pray that a bug, a disease, a germ, or sickness won't overtake the body while you're waiting for those stem cells to graft in. Most of us don't realize, and I certainly didn't, that a transplant really is just a small infusion. In a quite anticlimactic moment the nurse takes a tiny bag out of dry ice, hooks it up to an IV, and runs it right into the body. It is not a surgery, like we think of with an organ transplant. It is just a simple infusion of stem cells back into the body. That little bag, just a few inches big, literally is a life source to bring a person back to life. It's actu-

ally pretty amazing when you think about it. Surprised we had a party? I think not!

Radiation and the Party that is non-Medically accurate

For children, radiation treatments are pretty rare because of the significant long-term side effects. Depending on their age, some children will be sedated for their treatments (Emily was.) Overall, it was a pretty easy sedation. They would inject her with a white milky substance called "Propofol," which is a general anesthetic that would quickly put her to sleep and last just long enough to do her radiation, where-upon, when finished, she would wake up just as quickly. This became our morning routine for weeks. We'd get up early, go sit in the radiation department, do her session, and come home. Radiation made her very tired. I tried my best to creatively explain to her what was going to happen.

Here it goes.

I explained to her that one of the reasons we never knew "Tumor" was in her was that he was hiding. It had taken six months to find out why Emily was so sick. She knew she was sick. She knew she had fevers. She knew she had pain in her stomach. So she understood that we didn't know it was a tumor for a long time. I also explained that the tumor was

A Peek Into Our World
Bye Bye B.M.T. ~ The Freedom Party

Written July 4, 2010

When you have a child with cancer, every holiday is so momentous because in the back of your mind you always wonder, will my child be here next year to celebrate this? I think that's the one thing that really separates cancer moms from other moms. Most people don't ever think, "This might be my child's last birthday. This might be my child's last Christmas. This might be the last Halloween costume I ever purchase." Those thoughts aren't part of normal everyday life. But when you have a child with cancer, these thoughts seep into your subconscious, fight for space in your mind, and even if you fight them, you know they are there, lurking in the background wanting to scare you. You don't want to think that this could be my last Halloween, but you know in the depths of your soul that there is always that potential, that risk. You want every single holiday to be so important and special to capture memories that might be the last memories you'll ever have. I felt that way on the Fourth of July.

I wanted Emily to see fireworks. This little girl had just spent November until July Fourth confined inside a hospital, only occasionally getting a few days to escape and go home. I wanted her to experience an incredible Fourth of July. I couldn't take her out in public; she just had her bone marrow transplant and she couldn't be around people. That's when God puts angels in your life. Special people who just embrace you and your child more than you could ever imagine. That special angel came in the form of Jordyn Hollander. Jorydn is a friend of mine, a fellow East Coaster trapped in Denver. His loft overlooked Coors Field, which has a huge fireworks celebration. Unfortunately, he wasn't going to be there but offered his place for us to go to and watch the fireworks display from his private balcony. We drove to his loft, parked, and went upstairs. I was so excited! We were going to stand on his balcony, just the two of us, overlooking the beautiful firework display. Emily's first real "normal" experience in eight months!

She was tired. She crawled onto the couch.

"Stay awake, Emily." I said. "There's another hour before the fireworks."

She rested her head on the pillows.

"Stay awake, Emily, just another hour."

She closed her eyes.

"Emily! Emily, wake up!"

I stood alone and watched that beautiful firework celebration on the balcony while Emily lay curled up on the couch sleeping soundly not even disturbed by the sound of the fireworks bursting overhead. To my utter disappointment, afterwards I scooped her up, put her back in the car, and drove downtown to return Jordyn his key.

You know, sometimes, our biggest plans don't work out the way we planned. All our planning, preparation, and imagining what it will be like fizzle up into nothingness. But what did I want? I wanted a great memory of a Fourth of July with my daughter. Now I will always have the memory of Emily sleeping in that loft, all snuggled up, while fireworks were going off all around her. Remembering that she wasn't in a hospital and instead sleeping on a couch like a normal kid is a better memory than any firework show ever could be.

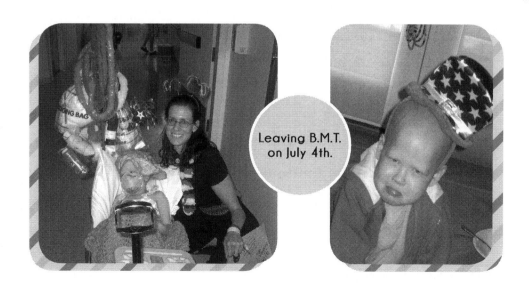

Leaving B.M.T. on July 4th.

hiding in her stomach, hiding behind her organs, hiding behind her kidney, hiding so nobody would know he was there making her sick. Now that she had kicked his butt out we never, ever, wanted him to be able to hide in her again. This was why we were going to do radiation.

When you think of radiation, what do you think of? Well, I thought of the sun and radiant beams of light. Keep in mind I had never actually seen radiation, nor had I ever actually witnessed what happens during a radiation treatment once they close the door. So my sun vision wasn't based on any medical understanding. I simply thought of radiation like a sun beam. So I told Emily that we were shooting beams of light into her, and it would light up her inside, light up her belly, so that if tumor ever tried to hide in her again her body would be able to see him right away. Her body would be able to spot him, and he couldn't sneak away and hide. I reminded her that she had bone marrow stem cells who would be ready to kick his butt after being at boot camp. There would be no way the tumor could hide in her again because her insides would now be lit up like the sun.

I also explained to her that her special bed would be her comfy pillow to lie in. So when they were doing her mold, it was to help make her a comfy pillow that she could lie on while she got her sun.

Emily will tell you that radiation was probably her favorite part of her cancer treatment because she got to take a nap every day. We became friends with the families that we saw every morning, day after day, coming to get their treatment. Emily was one of the few children in the room, with her little bald head dancing around.

I often wonder what happened to so many of those people, and I wonder if they wonder what happened to Emily? I pray they are miracles too.

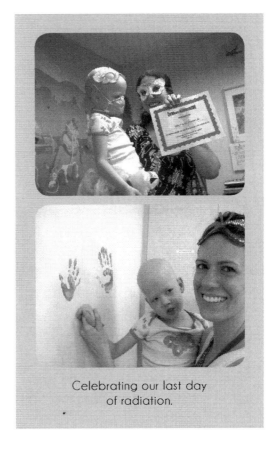

Celebrating our last day of radiation.

Parties Aren't Just For Cancer

During the course of Emily's treatment, the doctors discovered from her CAT scans that she also had a hole in her heart. It's called an Atrial Septal Defect, otherwise known as an ASD. We didn't even know it was there. It wasn't related to her cancer in any way; it was just another random thing that she was born with. They informed me that because it was so small it wouldn't really bother her right now. I could certainly wait and prolong getting it closed until she was older, but it was large enough that it would need to be closed eventually. I reasoned the best time to "fix" her heart would be after she was done with treatment, and she was cleared with her oncologist. I figured she was still friends with all the nurses and familiar with the hospital, and we were still in "medical mode." I didn't want to wait for a year or two, or maybe even three, and subject her to being brought back into the hospital yet again.

Six months after the end of treatment, we went back in for what we now call "The Butterfly Party." Why did we call it that? Simple: in order to close the hole in her heart the doctors would sedate her and stick a little device called a trans-catheter up through her leg, up into her chest, and then into her heart. The device would then open up and close the hole. It is the little metal device, the trans-catheter, that looks like a butterfly. It opens up on both sides just like little wings of a butterfly.

How did I explain to my 5-year-old what an Atrial Spetal Defect was and how a trans-catheter was going to close it? I made it fun of course. I told her that her heart had a little opening in it, and it was making her heart work harder than it needed to, and we needed to close that hole up. Her doctors were going to stick a little butterfly in her heart and make sure that all the blood was moving in the right direction. The little butterfly's wings would flap and make sure that her heart didn't have to work so hard. Since she had stem cells that went to Boot Camp, sun shine inside her tummy, and a Stupid Tumor who hid in her, a butterfly didn't seem that unreasonable.

I hope you're beginning to see how you can take ANYTHING your child is facing, use your imagination, and come up with a way to explain it that not only makes sense but is fun too! And your crazy explanation will usually lead you to an even more fun party. We got a butterfly net, and we wore butterfly wings. We even found in her closet a little outfit that had butterflies all over it. We brought rainbow colored streamers, plates and cups, and checked in for our butterfly party.

When Emily woke up from surgery, they brought her up to the 6th floor, which was not the oncology floor. The nurses didn't know us. They didn't know Emily, and they didn't know they were in for a party! Once we were in her room we had to decorate to make it fun! Now, we were only going to be there one night, but one night or not, we were there for a party! Since her surgery was pretty simple with little recovery, we were ready for a great time. One of my favorite memories was when her doctor walked in and there was my little 5-year-old sitting in her bed, and he said, "Wow! I've never seen such a decorated room," while eying up all the decorations and streamers.

Emily looked at him, quite sure of herself with her little hand on her hip and said, "Dude, did you think I was going to sleep in a boring room?" The look on her doctor's face was priceless.

An ASD was just one more excuse to have a party. That night, after she was feeling better, she went up and down the halls "flying" in her butterfly costume. We went down to the end of the hallway, all the way to the parent lounge, where she could climb up on the chairs and look out the huge windows to watch the twinkling lights of the Denver city skyline. We decided the view was so pretty we brought all her stuffed animals from her room down the hall and lined them up on the window ledge so they could take in the view too. We played Eye Spy looking out the windows trying to stump each other on what we could find. This might sound crazy, but compared to other hospital stays this was like staying in a hotel! Since she really wasn't "sick," it was really just a night away from home. Who knew you could take a mini "vaca" in a hospital?

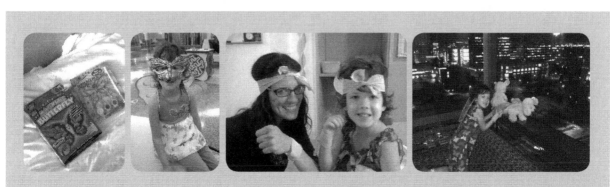

The Butterfly Party

Fun Factor

So, how do you plan the perfect party? It's a lot easier than planning a birthday, a sweet sixteen, a bar mitzvah, or a graduation party. In fact, it can be easy and more important, as any parent who is going through cancer treatment can appreciate, it can be cheap.

The first step is to determine what big milestone your child needs to complete over the next month, or three months, or six months. (We never planned more than one party at a time.)

- ✿ What is the next big milestone that your child would need to achieve?
- ✿ Is it completing a certain amount of medication?
- ✿ A number of rounds of chemo?
- ✿ Having a surgery?
- ✿ Is it going through some kind of surgical procedure?
- ✿ Maybe it's just reaching a milestone of the number of days you've been in the hospital, or even better, getting out of the hospital!

Whatever big event is coming up, that's your next party!

Our next big celebration will be because…

_____

_____

_____

_____

_____

Next, think of a theme. Sometimes our themes had to do with seasons, or times of year. For example, when we checked out of bone marrow transplant, it happened to be the Fourth of July, and we called it our "Freedom Party." We had a red, white, and blue theme, and we were FREE from B.M.T. Our October party was "Scare Cancer," simply because it was Halloween.

Below is a list of themes we came up with. Many times, Emily came up with a theme, or I would come up with a few and let her choose. You might think that you're not creative, but give your kid a chance. He or she might be more creative than you think! Ask other people. Go to Facebook and ask for suggestions, Themes and ideas are just endless. The older your child is, the more "into it" he or she can get coming up with unique themes. A lot of times, I would just go to the dollar stores and, depending on what the season was or what the upcoming holiday was, I would purchase whatever the store had out. For example, one time we did a Hawaiian luau theme because when I walked into the dollar store that's what was there! You could do a Valentine's Day theme or a good luck theme (St Patty's day!) It doesn't need to be seasonal; it could just be based on what your child is interested in. What's most important is that your party does not cost a lot of money. I would estimate that the average I spent on a party was $20 or less, costumes and all. We would try to find things that were already in our house that we could use.

Questions to Ask Yourself:
- ❀ What does my child like?
- ❀ What characters does my child like?
- ❀ Movie or TV characters?
- ❀ Favorite celebrities?
- ❀ Favorite sports?
- ❀ Favorite singers?
- ❀ A special hobby or interest?
- ❀ Are there any big milestones—a number of days, a number of treatments—coming up?

What major holidays are coming up around this next big event?

_____

_____

_____

_____

Don't worry if you can't come up with a fun catchphrase. I think we can stress ourselves out that we don't think we're creative enough to come up with a fun idea, but a lot of times, our themes will come from our kids themselves. The idea is to **HAVE FUN!** After all, who doesn't love a party?

Theme Ideas

Whip Cancer's Butt

Dress up as a little chef. Get a paper chef's hat from the party store and pair it with black pants and a white top. Use a wire whisk and pot holder from your kitchen. Talk about how a whisk is used to whip food, but you are "whipping cancer's butt!"

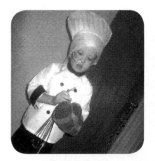
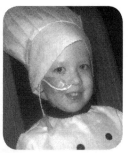

Make Cancer Walk the Plank

Get a paper pirate hat from the party store and a plastic sword. Most party stores have pirate themed plates, cups, and streamers. Explain how pirates would make people walk the plank, fall into the water, and die. Well, that's what you're going to do to cancer. In our case, Stupid Tumor was going to walk the plank, fall into the water, and die.

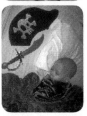
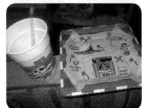

Put Cancer to Sleep

What girl doesn't love a princess? My gosh, you could build a whole year of cancer themes just around the Disney Princesses! Dress up like Sleeping Beauty and put cancer to sleep... for good.

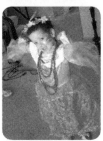

Scare Cancer

This works especially well if it's already around Halloween, and it's easy to find cheap Halloween decorations at the dollar store! Witches hats with hair are especially fun when you are bald! You could be a vampire and take a bite out of cancer. A wizard can put a spell on cancer. (If your child loves Harry Potter that could be another great theme.

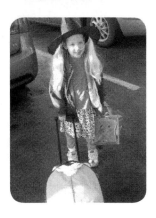

Theme Ideas

Wrap It Up

Perfect during the holiday season or for a last treatment hurrah! Use Christmas decorations you might already have, wear red and green, and use Santa hats and reindeer ears.

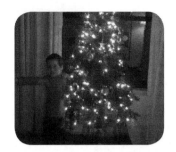

One Year, Let's Cheer!

We used this theme at her one year off treatment party. You could also use this to celebrate one year through treatment or one year post transplant etc. The party store has one-year-old birthday decorations and accessories. I actually found a great necklace that was pink and had glitter all over it at my local party store. It read: "Another Year of Fabulous." She wore the necklace with a pink skirt and pom-poms and pigtails! You could also use a Halloween cheerleader costume or you might even have one of your own!

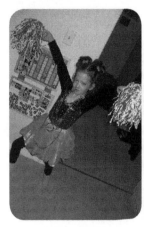
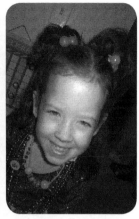

Flower Power

Decorate everything in flowers. Maybe a flower top, skirt, or dress. Use flower hair accessories and clips, (Hawaiian leis are perfect for this!) You could hand out fake flowers from the dollar store as party favors. Keep in mind most hospitals would not want you to bring real flowers to an oncology floor.

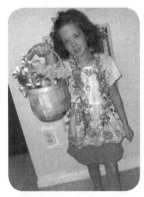
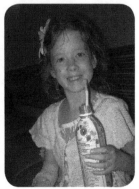

Scratch Cancer

An easy costume with Halloween cat ears and tails. You can draw on a nose and whiskers with black eye liner. Plus, it's even more fun to growl and roar like a tiger as your child pretends to scratch cancer so it will run away and hide!

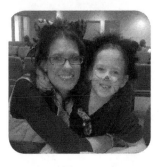

Theme Ideas

Erase Cancer

This was an Emily original. Yup, those are erasers I glued all over her! You can even hand out cute decorative erasers as party favors.

Too Cool for Cancer

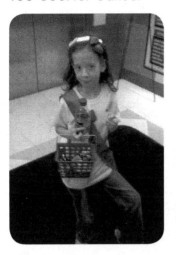 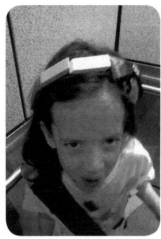 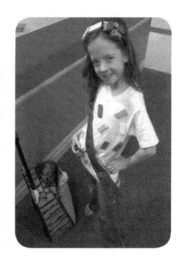

Dress in blue (or as Elsa from Frozen!) Wear sunglasses, snowflake accessories, or crystals. Draw snowflakes on with white eye liner. Hand out kid's party sunglasses or wintergreen mints as party favors. Dress in a scarf, gloves, and snow hat! Or, go in an opposite direction and wear a kid's leather bomber jacket, slicked back hair, and shades. (Think of the T birds from Grease!)

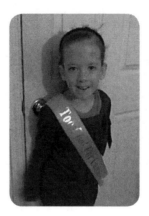 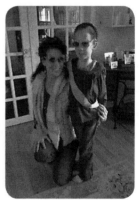

* Most of our themes came from costumes we already had at home in her costume box! Use what you already have or ask to borrow friends' costumes. Most people have a box of old Halloween costumes stashed away somewhere! Thrift stores can be a great resource too!

Helpful Hint

Often you will be waiting around for test or scans and be completely bored. During our "Too Cool For Cancer" party, we found ourselves stuck in a pre-screening room waiting for her MRI. It was taking longer than usual because they weren't sure if she would make it through the MRI without anesthesia. (It is hard to stay that still in something so loud and claustrophobic for so long!) We needed some entertainment, so we started dancing around our room, and we came up with a silly song:

"MRI!, MRI!
My Mommy does the Chi Chi Chi!"

Now I have no idea what a "Chi Chi Chi" is, but we needed something that would rhyme with MRI. (In my mind I pictured doing a Cuban Cha Cha!) The nurse (who didn't know we make cancer fun) opened the door in shock and said, "What are you doing in here?!?!" There was Emily, singing and dancing in her hospital gown as if it were a Friday night dance party.

As we left the hospital, my wise little Miracle Baby looked at me and said, "Cancer is fun if you make it fun." I asked her what her favorite part was, and she told me it was having a party and handing out sunglasses to everyone.

That is how my six-year-old views cancer follow up care: as fun. But she's right. And guess what? It's fun for me too. Being a single mom means most of the time I'm trying to take care of life. You

know, just the bustle and busyness of every day: working, grocery shopping, laundry, baths, homework, bed times. All those things that eat up our time. The biggest blessing of her follow-up treatment is that when we "Do Cancer" we "Do Cancer" and we don't "do" anything else. She gets 100% uninterrupted time with me. In an odd way these parties have been some of our most special times together because we're not busy doing all those other things. No taking emails, phone calls, or telling her to wait a minute. I am there, totally focused on her. I'd love to say in the real world it's like that all the time, but as a single mom it's not, and for Emily this is her mom time. Take that Cancer: we will find something to be grateful for even in our follow-up!

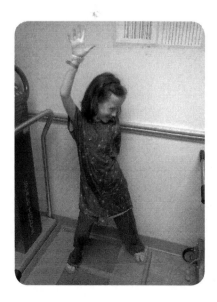

GUM, GIGGLES and GROSSNESS

Keep It Simple and Keep It Fun

Making Cancer Fun isn't always about the big parties and celebrations. It's really about finding the giggles in the day-to-day, the mundane: the puke buckets, lab draws, and endless hours living in a hospital room. That's what really made our experience different. In this chapter I'll share with you the small things that can have big impact. Not everything will be relevant to you and your child (depending on their age, treatment, symptoms, and side effects). Maybe just one or two ideas will resonate with you. That's okay. Remember, this book is not for you to use as a step-by-step guide and recreate what we did. It's to get you thinking like a kid again and come up with ways you want to face your child's cancer with fun. It's to inspire you to think of ways to shift the energy in your child's room from doom and gloom to giggles and laughter.

CHOOSING YOUR DAY

One of the hardest parts about being in the hospital is that children have no choice. They don't have a choice about what's going to happen to them. They don't have a choice about what they can eat. They don't have a choice about when they can leave their room. Sometimes they don't even have a choice about where they can go to the bathroom! I tried to find ways to give Emily as many choices as possible. Think about it. An adult who is sick, even in the hospital, has choices. We can take the doctor's recommendations or not. We can have the surgery or not. We can eat the recommended diet or not. Children don't have those choices because we, as their parents, make the decisions for them. Giving children choices gives them a sense of control. After all, here I am dealing with a 3-year-old who already wants to be the boss of the world and who is already going through the stages of finding her independence, and developing her own sense of self, and she is being denied monumental

> " A day without laughter is a wasted day.
>
> Charlie Chaplin "

childhood milestones, because she's being kept in a hospital, where all of her choices are being taken away from her.

In many respects, my choice was taken away from me too. There were only so many choices that I could make for her; a lot of it was beyond my control. I think that one of the hardest parts we had to struggle with was that we were really at the mercy of our doctors. We needed to listen to them from a place of trust, trust that they were going to do their best to take care of my child, and to trust their wisdom. Don't get me wrong, I am a huge believer in advocating for what you believe is right for your child. However, when it comes down to it, if she needed that surgery, she needed that surgery. If she needed that medication, and it was life-or-death, she was getting that medication.

i Get it, the Parent's Perspective:

Childhood cancer can feel like a roller coaster, especially when you are told one thing, but something else happens. I know, it happened with us too. Emily had formed a horrible blood clot during her treatment. As a result, she needed Lovenox injections in her legs—a blood thinner that would prevent a larger life-threatening clot

from forming. Worse yet, these injections were painful! She received her injections in her little thighs, rotating legs each week. In order for me to administer the injections at home, the nurses would implant an insulfon into her thigh each week. For us non-medical people, it's basically a needle that you stick into the leg, and it leaves behind a plastic tube so I could insert the needle and properly inject the medication into her leg. Each injection was painful, and she had to get them twice a day for months and months and months. Every time I would think, *"Okay, only twelve more weeks,"* the doctors would say that unfortunately the clot was still there. Finally, it got to a point where they just said, "She's going to need this for the rest of her treatment." As a parent, it was one of those moments when I felt helpless. I was angry because the doctors said it was only going to be twelve more weeks. Then it was only supposed to be two more months. Then it was only supposed to be four more weeks. Yet, now they were saying she was just going to need this for the rest of her treatment! Liars. I have to tell my baby I lied to her too. Her little legs, her teeny, tiny, skinny legs were so black and blue that even after treatment, it took months and months for the black and blue to go away. I thought those little yellow brown bruises would stay on her legs forever. It sure seemed like forever. That helpless feeling again, thinking, *"My child is being hurt, and there's nothing I can do."* Worse yet, in this case, I was the one doing the hurting. I had lost my control.

One small way I chose to take back some control was letting Emily decide what kind of day she wanted to have. On the back of the hospital room door, we would hang a piece of construction paper (one for each day), and we would write down what "type" of day we were going to have. Sometimes it was an animal theme day. (Ex: a monkey day or an elephant day.) Some days it was a feeling theme day. (Ex: a silly day or a laughing day.) She could even choose a color day. It was important that she didn't choose negative themes (a sad or angry day) because we didn't want a day like that. Sure, there were moments when she could choose to be angry, but not for an entire day.

Whatever she chose became the theme for the day. The creative part was incorporating that theme into everything we did. This is where getting the staff on board can make such a difference. For example, when she chose a monkey-themed day, everyone who came into the room had to act like a monkey when they first entered the room. Now most residents, they're young, they're in school, they're pretty cool with it. You do also get some of those serious surgeons, or doctors who have been around for a long time who don't want to act like a monkey.

Sometimes I would just say, "It's a monkey day! We really need you to you to act like a monkey." They didn't know what to say! When you are so over-the-top silly, people just don't know how to react. Politely ask: "I'm so sorry, but I just need you to act like a monkey for a minute before we can have that discussion, or before we can do that treatment, or before we can take that medication." Since we were at a children's hospital, most everyone, especially the nurses, were totally on board and happy to participate! Remember again, all of this is done to make their jobs easier. A cooperative, happy child is easier for everybody, including those serious doctors. You'll have some doctors that will be super fun (one of her doctors made the best monkey face ever!). Some of them get really into it! They love that you're being proactive and keeping your child's attitude in check. Some, you're going to have to work up a little bit. We'd ask them to act like a monkey, or to make their best elephant noise, or to do the silliest thing they could think of. For 3 or 4-year-olds to see their serious doctors, their serious nurses, all of a sudden make an elephant trunk and start snorting in the air can be hysterical, and even something fun.

Who was going to walk into the room? Who were we going to ambush with the day's theme? Who was going to be serious, who was going to do it, and who wouldn't want to participate? If they didn't participate, when they left we just said, "Poo on them. They are sooo not fun." Something so simple made our day fun! It was a small way that she could have control. We kept a whole door full of themes, and we would write what people did. Let's say you had to do something silly, we would have people write on the piece of construction paper what they had done that was silly. Maybe they hopped on one foot, or maybe they flapped their arms like a pelican, or maybe they sang a silly song, or maybe they pretended to pick their nose and roll their eyes. It didn't have to be something big, but just something silly they could do. We continued to try to find ways to make things fun, and we kept our papers hanging on her door, re-reading them, and laughing at all the fun things people had done.

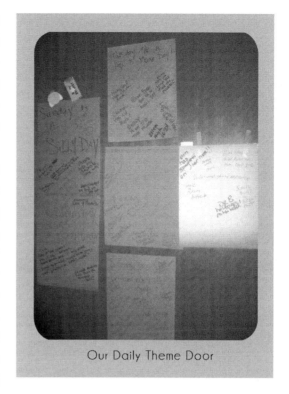

Our Daily Theme Door

tHe Puke CHaRt

There is a reason this chapter is called Gum, Giggle and Grossness, and I have to admit even the nurses thought this was disgusting, and it was, but Emily puked....a lot. If you have a sensitive tummy stop reading now. (Okay, we all know if you're in club cancer you get over your gross factor pretty fast, so....read on.) Emily had what they called "cyclical vomiting." That meant during her worst treatments of chemo (the dreaded Cisplatin drug) she would vomit every 15 minutes, all day and all night. She had acid burns running down her throat,

Fun Factor

Choose an **Animal Theme**: (Your child's favorite animal is a good place to start!)

_____

_____

How could you pretend to BE that animal?
(What sound does it make? How does it move? How does it eat?)

_____

_____

What is one funny thing you could create with that animal:

_____

_____

Choose a **Color Theme**: _____

What are some thoughts that come into your mind when you think of that color:

_____

_____

What is one funny thing you could create with that color:

_____

_____

Choose a **Feeling Theme**: _____

How do you act when you feel that way: _____

Now take that action and make it 10 times over the top more dramatic—how would you act then:

_____

_____

What other thoughts come into your mind when you think of that feeling?
(Maybe a silly story from your own life about that feeling?)

_____

_____

_____

down her little chin, on the outside of her, burning her skin. She was becoming raw, from having so much vomit. She would basically sit up, puke, lie back down for a few minutes, sit up, puke, lie back down. It was horrible. All the anti-nausea medications weren't working, and she was going to need a second round of this particular chemo. Because they were concerned about the long-term internal damage from that much vomiting, the hospital actually ended up approving her for a medication that normally is never used in children her age. I believe she was the first child under 7 to actually use it in the hospital, (which is why she needed her "special exam" with Molly and was later used as more proof of her Miracle Kid status.) The risk of the medicine was less. We're talking severe vomiting. And when she would puke, she would puke up all different kinds of things.

Emily also has a pickle addiction that started in the hospital. Now, I don't know medically what was going on that was causing my Miracle Kid to crave pickles, but that was all she wanted. I would bring her plates and plates of pickles. She would eat all those pickles, and she would proceed to vomit them all back up. You would think after this went on each time, she

would stop eating the pickles. I mean, I ate a yogurt once while I was sick, and I think it was three years before I could eat yogurt again. But not Emily. She didn't care if they came up as fast as they went in, she wanted her pickles. I began to call it "Pickle Puke," and we proceeded to make a

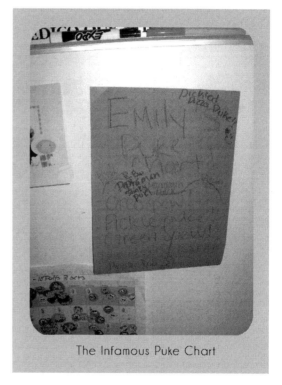

The Infamous Puke Chart

big chart in her room. Everything she would vomit up, we would look at the bucket of vomit and describe on the chart what it was that she puked. It could be pickle puke. It could be slimy, scum-sucking salami. It could be crumbly, chunky cookies. It could be whatever, but we would come up with bizarre and disgusting names for all her different types of puke.

Now, fortunately, I have a kid who loves gross stuff. The grosser, the better, and yes, she's a girl. So, for her to look through her puke, decide what it was, and write it down on the chart, well…she thought that was hysterical!

The rest of us were pretty grossed out by it. The nurses particularly thought I had lost my mind, but we kept her chart of puke. Looking forward to what we could add to the chart and how gross it would be the next time she hurled. Just one more way to keep cancer fun.

Fun Factor

What is your child's favorite food that they will probably puke up at some point?

_____

What adjectives describe this food? (Slimy? Dry? Sour? Creamy?)

_____   _____

_____   _____

_____   _____

What color is it? _____

What is the grossest way you could describe it? (Pretend you are a 5 year old!)

_____

_____

_____

WRaP UP YOUR diaPeR

We even made diapers fun. Emily was on a medication called Lasix, which would make her pee out all the water she was retaining. She was going through diapers and diapers and more diapers. For months, she looked like the Stay Puft Marshmallow Man all puffed out. As you can imagine, all that urine meant lots of diapers. Piles and piles of diapers. Constantly changing diapers and sometimes even layering more than one on to try to hold in all the urine. (Gross huh?) We also had to save all the diapers because the nurses would measure her input and her output to try to keep her fluid balanced.

Well, in true Making Cancer Fun style—always trying to find fun things to do in the hospital—one day I came back to her room with a roll of curling ribbon and markers. One thing that was great about Emily was how much she liked gross stuff. The grosser the better! She actually liked the surgeons the best because they got to deal with blood, guts, and gore. The nurses were second-ranked. They of course had pee, puke, and poop to deal with. Doctors, on the other hand, spurred very little interest because all they did was come into the room, talk, and leave. We were definitely blessed to have some amazing nurses taking care

of her. So, of course, when our nurses became like second family, we had to have fun with them too.

So one particular day when Emily was "filling up" a diaper, we took it off, and I pulled out some curling ribbon. She said, "What are we going to do?"

"Well," I said. "Let's make our diapers into presents."

We wrapped up her diaper like a present with a big bow and left it in the bathroom on the scale. We waited patiently to see what the nurses would do. Of course they thought this was funny! Eventually the wrapping diapers up into presents turned into to writing on them with markers. We would leave funny little notes and jokes for the nurses on her diapers to see how much we could make them laugh. Something as little as curling ribbon, pee, and markers can bring a little bit of sunshine into an otherwise pretty boring day.

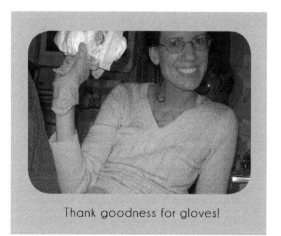

Thank goodness for gloves!

Fun Factor

What's your favorite joke?

_____

_____

_____

Is your child old enough to understand a riddle? Do you/they have a favorite?

_____

_____

_____

_____

Look up jokes and riddles online—there are tons of joke websites!
Write down your favorites:

_____

_____

_____

_____

_____

_____

_____

_____

_____

_____

_____

_____

Remember that you are in a children's hospital, so make sure your jokes are clean, G-rated, and non-offensive! This should be a no-brainer, but when you're a parent working on basically zero sleep and you are stressed to the max, it's just a friendly reminder!

Can You Relate? You Know You've Been at the Hospital Too Long When...

Written February 21, 2010 at 3:24am

In the shower last night at home while Em's tucked safely in bed at home...all of a sudden I think..."Oh no! Did I give the nurse my phone number?"

I open the drawer under my microwave to grab a spoon...because that's where they are in the hospital...note that is NOT where they are in my home.

I hear pumps beeping in my sleep.

I refer to the hospital as "the hotel."

POOPING ON a MONKEY'S face

Part of Emily's inpatient treatment consisted of having to keep track of her input and output. Yup. Tracking her poop. Consequently, she often had to poop in a "hat," which really consisted of a little white plastic tub-like thing that went over the toilet seat to catch her poop. Gross huh?

Emily didn't want to get out of bed to walk to the bathroom, much less poop on a toilet in some plastic white poop catcher. Remember though, there is always a way to make something fun. And what's more fun for a 3-year-old then pooping on pictures? I used Sharpie markers to draw funny images on the inside of the "hat" and then she would poop "on them." Ok, take the gross part out

of it, and that some psychotherapist might be appalled, and realize I am trapped in a hospital room begging a stubborn 3-year-old to get up, walk to a bathroom, and poop. Desperate times called for desperate measures. Time to poop on an elephant. A smiley face. A monkey. Now, I'm no artist—not by a long shot. If I were, my drawings probably would have been a lot more creative, but I am an improviser. I can match my 3-year-old's grossness with that of a frat boy, so a drawing I will make. I'm not sure why pooping on a monkey's face is funny to a kid, but it is. Part of the deal was that she couldn't see what I had drawn until she had gotten up out of bed and walked her way into the bathroom. (Curiosity might have killed the cat but it made my Miracle Kid walk.) What I learned is that the more ridiculous I made it, the funnier it was.

"Ewww no! Stinky!" The "monkey" would yell out as she pooped on him.

"Oh yummy I love to eat poop! Was that spaghetti you ate earlier today?" the elephant would say. Time to go barf now.

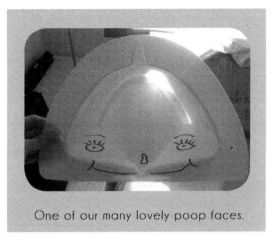

One of our many lovely poop faces.

Fun Factor

What are your child's favorite animals?

_____   _____

_____   _____

Does your child have a favorite superhero or animated character?

_____   _____

_____   _____

What would be the silliest thing that animal or character might say?

_____

_____

Does it have a certain type of voice it talks in (high, low, with an accent)?

_____

Continuing on the joke theme: if you have an older child maybe you write a joke instead. They can only find out what the joke is when they get out of bed and go to the bathroom. If they are too old to think pooping in a hat is funny, maybe you write the joke on the bathroom mirror with an erasable marker—something to get them curious enough to force themselves out of bed and into the bathroom!

the Right to Be angry

Now, sometimes, no matter how great our attitude is, we are angry and we're frustrated. Remember that a 5-year-old, or a 4-year-old, or any kid or teenager, does have the right to be angry. If we grown-ups are angry, for sure they feel just as angry. We can't penalize them, or make them feel bad for feeling angry. Sometimes we would make an angry sign. We would write down all the things that made us angry, and all the things that we didn't want to do. We listed all of the things that we hated about cancer, and things that we hated about Stupid Tumor.

We'd write them all down, hang it all up, and next to them, we would make a happy sign. I would ask Emily, "What are some of the good things about being here in the hospital?" One of the things that Emily put on her sign was that, "Mommy is with me all the time." Before her treatment, I was working. I was trying to get my life together after a horrific divorce, and it was hard to be

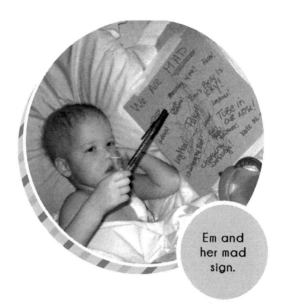

Em and her mad sign.

emotionally available for her all the time. I was emotionally, mentally, and financially drained. Some of the good things she felt about having to "do" cancer was I was not just physically there, but also emotionally and mentally with her as well. Trapped in a hospital room, I had no choice. There were no deadlines, work calls, or emails to return. It was just me and my Miracle Kid.

Another thing that made her happy was, "I finally get to choose what I want to eat every day." While that may not seem like a big deal, in a world where your body is poked, prodded, and peered at on a regular basis, and even your pee is monitored, getting to finally order whatever you want for each meal as if you were in a restaurant is an exciting sense of independence.

> " *For every minute you are angry, you lose sixty seconds of happiness.*
>
> *Ralph Waldo Emerson* "

Or it might be, "I get secret stash!" (More on stash later!) Reminding ourselves there are some good things about having to be at the hospital was important. We know what we focus on gets bigger, and focusing on the fun good things instead of just what we don't like changes our perception and heart to one of gratitude. Your mentality has to constantly go back to that age-old saying, "Every cloud has a silver lining."

tHe teasinG toe

Like all patients, when Emily was admitted into the hospital, the first thing the nurses did was hook her up to a machine to monitor her "vitals." They placed little stickers all over her chest to watch her heart rate, pulse, blood pressure, etc. and wrapped a thin bandage around her finger or toe to monitor her oxygen levels. Certainly, with living in Denver, oxygen levels were a big concern for a lot of patients (being in a higher altitude) but especially for Emily because her lungs weren't operating at full capacity. For months and months Emily lived with, slept with, and basically did everything but take a bath with a pulse oximetry (nicked-named a pulse ox) wrapped around her toe. Often the skin on her little toe would

grow raw from having that pulse ox wrapped around her for so long. And many times, she didn't want it there. She wanted it off! Sometimes we had to get a new pulse ox because the one she had was just so worn out. To make it fun I created the "Teasing Toe." The Teasing Toe was her left toe, the one that always wanted to wear the pulse ox, and when this toe got to wear the pulse ox, it would tease all the other toes.

"Nana nana boo-boo. Look! I get to wear the light! I get to wear the light!" it would tease. Of course, the other toes would cry, "No fair! No fair! We want to wear the light!" This was again another area where Emily got to be the boss. Emily got to be in charge and make the decision which big toe would get to wear the pulse ox. It was up to her which would be victo-

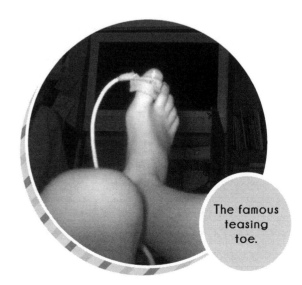

The famous teasing toe.

Fun Factor

What are the things that make your child most angry about being in the hospital?

_____   _____

_____   _____

_____   _____

How does that make them feel? _____

_____

_____

What are some of things about being in the hospital that aren't too bad? _____

_____

_____

Can you find the silver lining? (I know this one can feel hard.) What are some of the good things about being in the hospital? _____

_____

_____

Tips to Find the Silver Lining:

✤ Has your child had any visits from someone special?

✤ A present or gift they loved?

✤ Will they be a Make-A-Wish child?

✤ Has the hospital had any special celebrity or musical artist come visit that your child got to meet?

✤ What are some choices your child does get to make every day?

✤ A special nurse or doctor they especially like?

✤ Another oncology child they are now friends with who they otherwise wouldn't have known?

Force your brain to ask, "What can I be grateful for?" I know that's a sensitive question, but it was one I asked daily.

_____

_____

_____

_____

rious and celebrate and which would be defeated and crying.

"Em, which toe do you want it to be on today?" I would ask. She would make a huge deal out of getting to pick the perfect toe to wear the pulse ox. Of course, I would take her little feet, move them up and down, and talk as if I were her toes. "Pick me! Pick me! No, my turn! My turn! You had it yesterday! No! My turn!" Once we decided which toe was chosen the Teasing Toe would have the biggest fit. I remember Emily used to sit there, her legs crossed in her bed, wagging her Teasing Toe in the air. For a long time the Teasing Toe was like a member of the family, always

Fun Factor

What medical devices does your child need to use? Abroviac? A port? Pic line? Oxygen tube?

_____   _____

_____   _____

_____   _____

Can you give these devices a "life" of their own? What would their names be?

_____   _____

_____   _____

_____   _____

How would they behave? Would they be sassy or sweet? Demanding or whiny? Brave or scared? Think of them as if they were an over dramatic animated cartoon. Think like a KID!

_____   _____

_____   _____

_____   _____

teasing whether or not she would get to wear the light.

tHe GuM Buffett

When Emily was first diagnosed and had the chyle effusion (fluid around her lungs), she was put on a very strict low-fat diet. When that didn't help, her diet was scaled down to a no-fat diet, which was then scaled down to two juice boxes and two popsicles a day, which was further restricted to "NPO," meaning nothing by mouth. She wasn't allowed to eat or drink anything! Since she was receiving total parenteral nutrition (otherwise known as TPN) through her IV, the doctors weren't worried about her from a nutritional standpoint. But imagine being told you can't eat anything at all no matter how hungry you are. Not even a sip of water. Since the TPN was administered through an IV and not her stomach, she was hungry all the time. It was horrible. She would cry and scream and beg that she was hungry and would I please feed her. That her throat hurt her, and could we at least get her ice chips and even then the ice chips had to be rationed off. Even though I knew it was necessary, it felt like I was torturing my child. So in true Making Cancer Fun style, we created the Gum Buffett (since gum was the one thing that was allowed!)

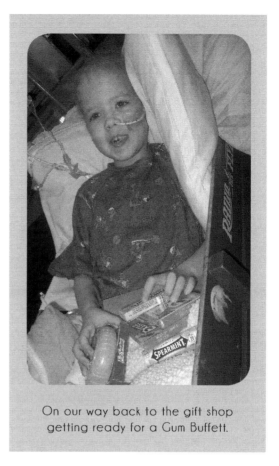

On our way back to the gift shop getting ready for a Gum Buffett.

Emily would get loaded into her little red wagon, IV pole and all, and we would take a trip down to the gift shop. There, right in front of us, in a huge display rack, were piles and piles of gum choices. Emily would take her time carefully choosing through the different flavors of gum. After making her selections, we would load her wagon up with gum and wheel back upstairs to her room. I would prop her back up in bed and in front of her place her buffet of gum.

Really, she would only chew each piece maybe a couple of times, but she would proceed to have her "dinner" of gum. I think it was the emotional feeling of chewing and eating "food," and experiencing the flavors of the gum, that calmed and soothed her most. After all, she was getting fed intravenously, so her body physically had the nutrients it needed. But not being able to physically eat, to have her stomach empty and rumbling, she decided gum chewing fit the food craving bill. Friends started sending gum in different flavors (Juicy Fruit became her favorite), and we would

Fun Factor

If your child is on a restricted diet, what CAN they eat?

_____   _____

_____   _____

_____   _____

How many variations and ways to make that food can you think of?

_____   _____

_____   _____

_____   _____

Can you make the food fun?

☆ Cut breads or vegetables into shapes with cookie cutters?

☆ Can you add food coloring into any foods to make them "silly" (blue mashed potatoes, purple oatmeal?) *Check with the doctor first on any diet restrictions.*

☆ Make pizza faces using vegetables for eyes, a nose, and a mouth.

☆ Make spaghetti mountains! Sing the song "On Top of Spaghetti" while you roll the meatballs off and make up stories about where the meatballs would roll to if they rolled out of your room. What adventures they would have in the hospital?

☆ Maybe your food fights with each other. Carrots argue about who is going to get eaten first. Who is "oranger?" Who is tastier? Have each one beg, "Pick me! Pick me!" Let your child choose the "winning carrot."

accumulate mountains of wadded up gum all from the gum buffet.

Goal Posters

Have you ever made a goal poster? Or created a vision board? Depending on your line of work, you may or may not be familiar with goal posters. I come from the direct sales world where goal posters are a way of life. Personal Development 101: make a goal poster. It gives us something to strive for and to focus on. Find a win! When you're "doing" cancer, every win counts. Emily knew I had goal posters, and now it was time for her to make her own. Some goals were easy—they were benchmarks for her cancer treatment. Six rounds of chemo, surgery, B.M.T., radiation, immune therapy, finish treatment, etc. Other goals were personal ones that she set. Go on a picnic, go back to the indoor rec center pool, visit New Jersey to see family, etc. One of her biggest goals was to sleep in a bear cave. That's what we called sleeping under the dining room table in our home when we covered it with sheets and made a little cave inside. What's funny is we only did this once, but it was just a few days before she was admitted to the hospital. My guess is that the "bear cave" almost became symbolic

for life without cancer to her. We had that bear cave on her goal poster for a few years before we finally did it again. (Truth be told, I woke up that morning with pain in parts of my body I didn't even know I had from sleeping on the floor, so I wasn't too anxious to achieve that goal again. I kept putting it off, but she was persistent!)

You might notice unless I'm talking specifically about your superhero Miracle Kid fighting cancer (and making it fun!) we usually referred to it as "doing" cancer. If you're wondering why there's a very specific reason for that.

Google defines "Fight" as: to take part in a violent struggle involving the exchange of physical blows or the use of weapons; a violent confrontation or struggle

Your Dictionary defines "fight" as: to face something and struggle through it

The Merriam-Webster Dictionary defines "do" as: to bring to pass

Your Dictionary Defines "do" as: to accomplish an action

Which energy feels lighter? Easier? Violence and struggle or accomplishment and passing? Our words create our reality, our feelings, and the energy around us. My daughter had to "do" cancer. She needed to face it and accomplish completing it. Yes, looking back at what we went through, it was a FIGHT. She fought for her life, and she won. I don't want to take away from that huge accomplishment. Of course we struggled, and some days she was at her worst, beat up physically by cancer. But I wanted to create less of that, not more. So I chose my words, the words that filled her room, life-giving words, carefully.

Making a goal poster is easy. All you need is poster board and a Sharpie. If your child is young, he or she could help draw pictures of the goals too. You can make a goal poster for daily goals (brush teeth, get out of bed, take medicine, do your physical therapy, etc.) and you can make one for larger goals. In B.M.T., the staff gave Emily a small goal chart that every day had a list of all the things she had to do. (My guess is that this was also partly for the sake of the parents to remember everything medically they had to do each day!) She would get to put a sticker next to each task she completed. Get ready to goal set!

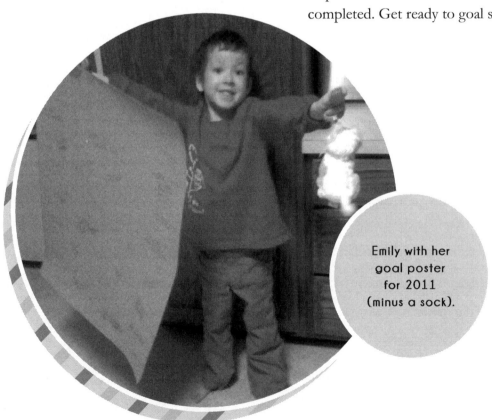

Emily with her goal poster for 2011 (minus a sock).

Fun Factor

What are the main benchmarks your child needs to complete in the next year for treatment?

_____   _____

_____   _____

_____   _____

What are some activities your child did BC (before cancer) that they want to go back to doing? Did they play a sport? An instrument? What clubs were they in at school? Were they in a Scout program or youth group?

_____   _____

_____   _____

_____   _____

Where are some places your child wants to go to? A favorite restaurant? Movies? Favorite local attraction? Favorite park?

_____   _____

_____   _____

_____   _____

Who are some people your child wants to see?

_____   _____

_____   _____

What are some experiences your child wants to have or be able to attend? A school dance? An important family holiday? A special vacation?

_____   _____

_____   _____

_____   _____

Most of the goals on your goal poster should be within a reasonable amount of time. The idea is for your child to have wins. Usually a goal poster should be for 1 year, so depending on their treatment setting goals for 6 to 12 months might be ideal. There can be a few long-term goals (finish treatment, go back to school, etc) but if all the goals are long term that takes away from the smaller wins.

If there are activities you know you know your child might not be able to do again try to keep these off the poster. We want the poster to be a positive motivation not a reminder of how different life might be after cancer. (Example if your child was an athlete but has had to face amputation maybe the goal is to join the Special Olympics not their competitive soccer team again.)

affirmations

It has been said that what we feed our minds has an impact on the reality we experience. How do you feed your mind? What are the thoughts that fill your mind each day? What are the affirmations that you tell yourself regularly? Everything, down to decorating Emily's room, was about creating positive affirmations. People from all over the country were sending me cards: people from my Mary Kay family, and my theater family, as well as my high school and college friends who had started following us on Facebook. Her room looked like a Hallmark store had blown up. Literally, floor to ceiling the walls were covered with cards. I would hang all the cards that people would send from across the country in front of her, and I would tell her, "Emily, these are all the people who are cheering you on, praying for you, and supporting you. They know you're a Miracle Kid, and they don't like Stupid Tumor either." I wanted her to feel she was surrounded by the love of so many people who cared about her. Sometimes we would take time to go through the cards, and we would read them again and again, to remind her of all the people who cared about her and all of the people who knew she was important and were praying for her.

One day, months into Em's treatment, a friend of mine, Yvette Alexander, showed up at the hospital. She had just taught a workshop on the power of affirmations, and she had printed out sheets of pink affirmations. She brought them to the hospital and said, "Here. I think you guys could use these." We hung those affirmations all over Emily's room. What you feed your mind and your spirit matters.

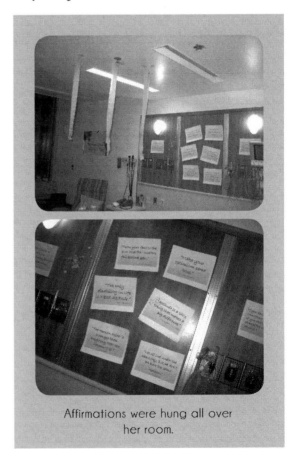

Affirmations were hung all over her room.

Fun Factor

Affirmations are used to reprogram our negative thought patterns to change the way we think or feel about something.

You and your child can create affirmations together, or you can create them and have your child decorate the paper.

✱ Your affirmations should be written in the present tense.

✱ Affirmations are always in the first person. Use "I am" and "My."

✱ Keep your affirmations short so they are easier to remember.

✱ Use emotion words. The more your affirmations connect with your feelings/energy the more effective they are.

✱ Don't use phrases like "I want" or "I need" because they are actually negative.

✱ Frame everything into the positive. Avoid words like can't, won't, and don't.

Examples:

Correct	Incorrect
I am so excited I finished my last round of chemo and am done with cancer!	When I finish my last round of chemo I want to be done with cancer.
I am strong and healthy.	I don't want to be sick.
I am a strong and healthy Miracle Kid.	I will be a strong healthy Miracle Kid.
I am crazy happy to be cancer-free!	I can't wait to be cancer free.

A Peek Into Our World ~ We're Still Makin' Cancer Fun & Now the ER Nurse Even Said So!

Written April 10, 2010 ~ 5 months into treatment

I've had two people tell me I make cancer fun. I am not sure if this is more out of shock and disbelief or out of sincere appreciation for my now full-time job as childhood cancer fun maker. Em was admitted to the ER today for puking (every 20 min since 2 am) and because she spiked a fever on the way over, 101° admits her and she's 104° right now, sleeping as I type this. She was lying in her little ER bed, miserable, puking, and shivering. I started pulling her stuffed animals out of her clinic bag to show her who came with us. The clinic bag helps make coming back to the hospital "fun." I fill it with toys and try to put in some secret new ones. Today, though, she was too sick to care.

Except when I pulled out our friends "the animals." A My Little Pony had made the "cut" into the bag, a cute giraffe was our new friend, and then there was Wilber the pig. I explained to Emily that as I was packing up her clinic bag at home all her stuffed animals were begging me to pack them, "Pick me! Pick me! No me!" they screamed from the big bin in the soon-to-be-play- room that is now currently referred to as the front- room, which for too long has been the nothing-room.

"And then..." I said, "Do you know what happened? Wilber jumped out of the toy bin and jumped into your clinic bag and wouldn't let anyone else go! He said he was a "master cruiser," and it had been too long since he was at the hospital, and he was going...and all the other animals were sooo jealous! THEY wanted to come too!"

Now all this was explained with Wilber jumping and hopping all over her ER bed, with frantic and exaggerated gestures on my part, while the ER nurse was setting up some kind of fluid. I then assembled all the animals on the side of her bed, hooked over the edge, looking over at her. Em, even in her pathetic, sickly, pukey, stinky state found Wilber's antics very amusing. "You are one fun mom," the RN said to me. "Well," I replied, "What else can you do with cancer?"

This sentiment was previously expressed by the radiation guy. Em and I were in there one day last month, getting yet another CAT scan, with our zoo full of animals. Of course our animals are always crazy in the CAT scan room. Moose tries to sneak through the donut while no one is looking, and I'm always having to pull him away from the machine. Pup or Wilber are always showing off how many times they've each been down for scans. Or the rookie animal who is in awe of their "first time" in the radiation room is checking everything out! I am also always jealous, of course, that Emily gets to go in the donut, no matter how many times I ask they just never seem to let me. "No Fair!" I regularly complain. And, of course anything that is "No Fair" to Mom is automatically very funny & cool to a 3-year-old.

So, upon our last visit to CAT the radiation guy says, "I don't think I've ever seen anyone make cancer as much fun as you two." That's probably the biggest compliment I've gotten since we've been here.

I hope that when Emily looks back on this time in her life, she won't remember the pokes, the 104° fever she has tonight as the nurses come in every 30 minutes to monitor her, and we're still in wait mode to see if she'll get transferred down to the PICU. She won't remember that damn leg med or the fact that the hospital overlooked giving her a narcotic before replacing her nose tube on Monday and I was livid. No, I hope she'll hear the word "cancer" and instead of the feeling of dread most of us associate that word with she'll think, "Hey that was fun...I cruised, I had parties, and I grossed my mom out daily. Cancer was cool." Maybe, just maybe, it will teach her to embrace all the pitfalls of life with laugher and silliness. Then again, after this, the kid deserves a break. I think she should get a pass on the "pitfalls of life." I hope you're taking note up there Big Guy!

THE SECRET OF SECRET STASH

Shhh... Don't Tell

One of the most fun things we did during treatment was what I refer to as "Secret Stash." When Emily was first diagnosed, everybody was quick to bring lots of presents, gifts, and stuffed animals. I was abundantly blessed with so many people generously giving to us. At times, it was overwhelming how many presents she was receiving, and it got to a point where she didn't really appreciate or value the presents, simply because she was inundated with them. Particularly because when she was diagnosed in November we were going into the Christmas season, so every non-profit, charity group, and organization was coming to the hospital on almost a daily basis, bringing toys and gifts for the children. Even for a person who doesn't have a huge circle of influence, if they're in a hospital setting, there are going to be a lot of opportunities for children to receive gifts and presents from organizations like Make-A-Wish Foundation, Toys for Tots Program, The Amanda Styles Cirelli Foundation, and the list goes on. I wish I had realized sooner, rather than a little more than halfway through her treatment, that she really didn't play with or appreciate all these different presents.

What I started to do instead when people would give us presents is say, "Thank you so much. I'm going to put this in her secret stash." I got a huge plastic bin, and I started filling it with all the toys and presents that we were receiving, whether it was through the hospital, through friends, or through a fundraising program, and I started stashing the toys away. Rather than her receiving lots and lots of presents that she didn't even play with, and barely looked at or tossed aside, I would just stash them. This way, when there were times she was bored, or when she didn't have a new present or something to entertain her, I could go to the secret stash and pull out a great gift.

This also became even more important as she started

> "I don't trust anyone who doesn't laugh.
>
> Maya Angelou"

getting out of the hospital and started going back and forth. In a lot of ways, I think it was actually easier staying in the hospital, than it was going back and forth. Once you're there, and you're immersed, you just start to live there. You get into what I call "hospital mode." You dress like you're at the hospital, you have all your personal care items at the hospital, you've moved in like it is a hotel room. Suddenly, you start to forget what the real world is like. It's such a mental shift, you begin to forget what it's like on the "outside." Fortunately, at 3 years old it was easy to forget what it was like outside; the hospital became her world. When she got to go home, though, that was different. She got to have multiple days of being at home, waking up in her own bed, going back to sleep in her own bed, and being able to sleep without a nurse coming in, poking her, prodding her, and drawing blood. She got to go without having X-Rays done every day, people coming in and out of her room, and eating cafeteria food. Instead, she got to eat food out of our kitchen. She got to get up and walk around. Even though it was hard, she got a taste of what the real world was like again.

Every time she came back to the hospital, especially because she knew she was going to get checked in to sleep there, it became harder and harder. When she went in for her Bio-therapy we would check in for five days, and she would know that she was going to have to stay there. And as soon as they would hook her up to those machines, hook in those IVs, she would be so angry, so combative, and so sad, because she knew her freedom was being taken away again. She knew that she was going to be sick, that she might be vomiting, and that she might have pain. Her type of Bio-therapy was so painful. They literally hooked my kid up to a narcotic the very first day. Everyone knew the treatment was painful, and even at 4 years old, she knew what those wires meant. She knew what that IV meant.

So, I controlled the only thing I could. I could make it fun. I could bring the Secret Stash. The night before I would fill up her rolling backpack with special treats and gifts that she hadn't seen before. Sometimes I would include some special toys, games, or books that she liked from home. But I would also always include a handful of new things. She loved crafts, and that always gave us something to do while sitting there bored in the hospital. The best gifts were ones that kept her entertained while she was going to be at the hospital, whether it was painting, drawing, coloring, or something she could put together, like mosaics. Even games, cards, or anything that was an activity we could do together was a winner. Depending on the child's age, of course, Mad Libs, DVDs, or cartridges for their gaming systems are also great.

While she was going through treatment I wasn't really working, so I didn't have any sort of budget that would allow me to go out and purchase a lot of fun things every time she went back to the hospital, especially since she was going once a month! This was why her secret stash became so invaluable. I could go to that box, pop in different prizes and presents and stash them away for her next in-patient treatment.

It became another fun thing about cancer. She would look forward to Secret Stash. She would ask, "Did you pack my Secret Stash? Mommy, make sure you get my Secret Stash." Now, the rule was she couldn't look at it until we got into the hospital and settled into our room. In the morning, she would get her backpack, but she couldn't open it. We would put it in the car. She would try to guess or get clues out of me, and I would never tell her. I'd say, "We have to wait until we get to the hospital."

It wasn't just getting to the hospital either. It was getting checked in, getting the ID bracelet on, getting to our room, meeting our nurses and getting settled; only then could she start to go through her Secret Stash. It became a way to make something that was really unbearable, bearable. It gave her something to look forward to when we had to check in.

Now, she goes to the hospital mostly for day visits. Scan, check ups, lab work, and such. During these routine visits there's always lots of downtime. Lots of sitting around waiting for a doctor or a test result or drinking contrast before a scan. Now, it's not a bag full but maybe one or two new

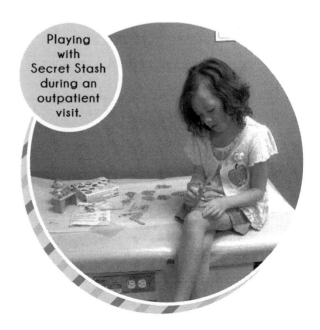

Playing with Secret Stash during an outpatient visit.

books, a new coloring book, or something that we can bring with us to do while we're waiting. But there's always something to look forward to.

Unintentionally, it also became useful when she was finally done with treatment and had to go back into the "real world" and have babysitters. Understandably, she wasn't used to being separated from me. She was used to my being with her all the time in the hospital, and we went through a period of separation anxiety. Giving her some Secret Stash to do with her babysitter was something she started to look forward to when she was separated from me, and it helped ease the transition. Like everything, it's always about trying to find the positive and the fun in every situation.

Fun Factor

Determine where you will hide the secret stash. A plastic bin? An empty drawer? A laundry basket? Try to avoid your child seeing the gift beforehand.

Helpful Hint: If someone brings a present, intercept it at the door. Explain to them about Secret Stash, then hide the gift. Still tell your child "Aunt Susie" brought a gift so they can thank them, but let them know "Aunt Susie brought you Secret Stash" so they know they aren't getting their gift now.

If possible, write a note on the gift so you know who gave it. Later, when you give your child their "stash" you can take a photo of him or her with the present and send it to the giver. This way the gift giver doesn't miss out on the enjoyment of seeing your child with their presents.

When you are out and see things on sale, add them to your stash. Dollar stores, Target dollar bins, and Michael's craft stores have great cheap gift bins. Sales after holidays can offer huge discounts as well.

Check out local kid's consignment sales and yard sales, but make sure anything you buy second-hand can be thoroughly cleaned and sanitized.

A Peek Into Our World ~ Emily Is a Pack Rat

Emily is a pack rat, and she has been since the time she could pack. It drives me crazy that Emily takes every toy she owns and stuffs them in bags until the seams are bursting. Then she'll ask me to find a specific toy that I have to search through bags and bags just to find. It also creates a huge mess...piles and piles of toys and stuffed bags. I just spent a week putting together a play room and neatly organizing all of her toys. All doll toys in the big basket, all crafts in the craft closet, all balls in the ball bucket, plastic food in the food crate, small miscellaneous toys in the big plastic bucket that has no name because what the hell is that plastic toy for anyway?

Tonight, the night before Emily's BMT admittance, I am packing my bag for a week at the Children's Hospital. I am packing her "clinic bag" (aka Secret Stash), I am packing my work bags for two appointments I'll hold before I get back to my house, and I'm packing party supplies for tomorrows BMT party. I hope the hospital is prepared for us, although they should have caught on by now that we look for any excuse to party. Emily is packing...bags and bags and bags. Who knows what's in half of that pile of mess. I grimace as my neatly arranged toys are pulled out one by one and stuffed into black holes of bags. I tell myself not to worry. After tonight, Emily won't be home for 100 days. I can unpack all those stuffed bags and reorganize all her toys, and it will be a full 100 days before she messes it up again.

And then I am overcome with guilt. My heart aches, and I know in that instant I would give anything, pack any bag, stuff any black hole, rip every toy of the shelf and throw it into the middle of the floor and let it stay there forever piling higher and higher until we had to climb over the pile to get into the room....to have her home, to have cancer gone, and to be at home, listening to her sort and pack her toys in the room next door, I am jealous of every mom I know with a messy house tonight. Do they realize how lucky they are to pick up toys? I will never look at a stuffed bag again and grimace. I will be thankful she's home to stuff them. And so, I think to myself...pack away little one.

WHEN it POPS UP, WHAT POPS OUT?

What To Say When You're On the Spot

Thinking on your feet takes practice, and coming up with something fun on the spot can feel daunting. Let me share with you a few scenarios where I had to make it fun on the spot. Since every child's cancer experience is different you may not be able to copy them directly, but you can get an idea of what it looks like when you are Making Cancer Fun! Think about how you can turn these ideas into ones that will work for you. Use the tips you have already learned including Yes…and. Try not to over think, just respond. What will make you a great improviser is that you don't think too much. If it pops into your head, it pops out of your mouth. Now, that may not be great when you're at work, dealing with your significant other, or need to talk to a medical professional, but when it comes to Making Cancer Fun, the less thinking the better. It's the one time you don't need to "think before you speak."

NO, MY MOM CAN'T SIT ON A PRINCESS PILLOW!

Written April 11, 2010 at 2:26 a.m. just 5 months into Emily's treatment

Em went for an X-ray today while in the ER. Well, actually three X-rays to be exact. Poor, miserable, neutropenic, fever running, puking, nauseated kid had to lay on an X-ray table for three belly pics, wearing a mask so no one could spread their disgusting germs on her and to keep her safe from those small grimy, grubby, cesspool filled broods of children running around the ER. (Funny how cancer makes you view once adorable, sweet, delightful children as dangerous microorganisms of filthy germs that are to be avoided at all costs).

> "
> *Humor is a universal language.*
>
> *Joel Goodman*
> "

Here's a peek into how it went:

"Em!" I exclaim. "Do you see the Princess Pillow???" The "princess pillow" is this big square block thing that is covered in a baby blanket that she sometimes has to sit on to get her X-rays.

She looks.

"Em! Do you think you're going to get to sit on a Princess Pillow?!?!" I ask in disbelief. "Is she going to sit on the Princess Pillow?" I ask the X-ray guy with a look of you-better-catch-on-quick-my-kid-is-sitting-on-that-damn-square-thingy-and-yes-it's-a-princess-pillow.

"Uh, yeah, she can sit on it," he says and brings it over.

I hop up on the X-ray table.

"Em! Do you think I could sit on a Princess Pillow?" I ask excitedly.

The X-ray guy looks at Em, "Do you want your mom to sit on a Princess Pillow?" he asks in a tone that makes me realizes he fully expects to get a "yes" and has yet to fully catch on to our game.

Now the kid who has not said a word in probably two hours since we got there, and has a look of complete exhaustion and miserablenesss, gets a stone cold look of determination and assertiveness in her eyes. They narrow. She stares right at the X-ray guy and shakes her head in an under-no-uncertain-terms, "NO!" as in, "No, only I get to sit on the princess pillow, ha ha ha aren't you jealous?"

Ahh, she'll be ok. She's still got her spunk.

Miracle Mike

Emily had a broviac for most of her treatment (an implanted IV). Once we started doing follow-up visits, her broviac was removed, and she was actually physically having to get "a poke," and it became a lot more traumatic. What sounds like a simple blood draw could result in screaming and me having to physically hold her down. Of course, the more she screamed and the more upset she would get, the faster her veins would collapse, and that would involve multiple pokes. The one good thing was we always saw Aileen, the same lab tech every single time. I told Emily Aileen only saw the Miracle Kids because she was the best of the best, and everyone wanted to see her, but only the very special kids got her for their nurse.

We were used to our routine. Comfortable, familiar, stable. Until that one fateful day when we checked in…(dramatic pause)…and learned that Aileen was not there! Apparently, she was out sick and, instead, some unknown "Mike" would be taking her spot.

Here's a peek into how it went:

Emily stood there, her eyes growing wide, I could see her thoughts racing. "Where is Aileen?" "Who is this Mike?"

As I watched the look of fear that began to overtake her, I looked at the receptionist and said quickly, "You mean Miracle Mike?" Again, all those years of improv taught me to think on my feet.

The receptionist looked at me confused and said, "Excuse me?"

I quickly shot back, "You mean Miracle Mike?" (Nodding my head in a "Please go with me on this" sort of way.) "Miracle Mike the one that we've heard about, but nobody's ever seen? We heard that since he only takes the very, very special Miracle Kids, no one actually gets to see him anymore. He's going to be the one drawing Emily's blood?"

She looked at me with a blank stare, and when I realized she wasn't catching on, I simply said, "Oh my goodness. We're so excited!" and moved Emily away.

Emily and I sat down, and I said, "Em did you hear that? It's Miracle Mike!"

"Who's Miracle Mike?" she asked skeptically. I quickly explained to her that Miracle Mike was the best of the best; he was the one all the kids wanted, but that he was only here for certain times. Word must have gone around the hospital about her coming today, and that since she was a Miracle Kid she was going to have Miracle Mike who was even better than Aileen!

I was so excited, my eyes were wide, my anticipation great. I couldn't wait to meet him! I'd only ever heard about him, never actually saw him in person! Emily started to get excited too. Who exactly was this Miracle Mike?

When Miracle Mike stepped into the waiting room and said "Emily Grace?" I jumped up and said with an abnormal amount of excitement for a mom in a clinic waiting room, "Are you Mike?"

He responded "Yes," and I continued with, "Miracle Mike! We've heard so much about you! We're so excited that you're doing her lab draw today. We heard Aileen wasn't here, and you're taking all of her miracle patients." With my eyes knowingly looking at him nodding my head in order to get him to go along. I said, "We've heard how great you are and that you do the best pokes in the whole hospital! We're so excited that you're getting to do our lab draw today. Emily look, It's Miracle Mike!"

He looked at me blankly and replied completely deadpan, "I have no idea what you're talking about." I realized at this point that he was not the sharpest tack in the box and proceeded to ignore him.

Well, it turned out Miracle Mike was not, in fact, a miracle. Two IV attempts later, and after pokes in both arms there was still no placement. So much for Mike. He called in another nurse who then proceeded to try to put the IV into Emily's wrist while she screamed, and still no placement. By now there were hysterics to the point she could barely breathe, and we needed to take a trip to the refreshment station for a drink and a break. We finally found one of our favorite nurses, Brandy, who calmed Emily down enough to get the IV into her other wrist.

Afterwards Emily and I agreed. She questioned, "Mom, I don't understand. I thought that was Miracle Mike?" I replied, "Em, I have no idea, but Miracle Mike was definitely not a miracle." Sometimes things just don't go as planned. But you keep going, keep smiling, and start looking for your next moment of fun!

tylenol Wars

Written June 19, 2010 In-Bone Marrow Transplant

Em doesn't want to take her Tylenol because her throat hurts. Her CAT scan showed her esophagus is inflamed, and they think the inflammation is all the way up to her mouth. So, I get it. It hurts. She's puking up blood. Her face is swollen. Her intestines are swollen, and they don't know why. Blood work normal, poop scoop normal, and we're waiting on one other test. Last night her temp was 105.9°. Today she is at 102.8°. The kid needs Tylenol.

How does one explain to a 4-year-old why she has to take this med that is going to burn her mouth that's filled with open sores making it harder to swallow? Our body is wired to steer clear of pain, and here I am, her mom, saying do it anyway even though, to quote Sara McLachlan, "This is gonna hurt like hell."

Well, here is my 9:30 a.m. fly by the seat of my pants shot....

I climb into bed with Em. She's lying on a cooling pad, with a wet cloth on her head. She looks at me with her blood-stained lips and swollen chipmunk cheeks.

"Em you feel crummy, right? Your body feels achy and tired, right? You want to know why?

Remember you got your stem cells and they got back from "boot camp" where they were learning to kick cancer's butt. Remember the BMT. chemo killed off all your white blood cells just in case there were any "traitors" in there, right? And your stem cells started making new baby white blood, remember? And then they became grown up white blood, right? And remember how you were surprising everyone because you had baby white blood before you were supposed to, right? And remember how on your chart you were only supposed to have this much white blood (I take my fingers and show a small 1 inch with my thumb and finger) and you had THIS MUCH (I spread my hands apart showing a big space) and even your doctors didn't know how you were doing it!! And it's because you're a Miracle Kid that your white blood is sooo strong!

Well, here's the deal Em, you got a buggy in your intestines. Do you know what your intestines are? You know how your belly hurts? (She nods.) Well, when you have food it goes in your mouth down all the way to your stomach and then into your intestines and then you poop it out. (Bringing up poop always a big hit—meanwhile I'm tracing my body from my throat all the way down—yes to my butt!) Well, your intestines have a buggy in there, a buggy who is friends with your tumor. Now your doctors are giving you antibiotics in your "tree" (IV pole) to help kill the buggies. But here's the deal, you are soooo strong and your white blood is

soooo strong that they're fighting the buggies off. So, your white blood ran down to your intestines and is having a war with those buggies! GET OUT OF EMILY! POW POW! GET OUT OF EMILY GRACE, MIRACLE KID! And they are all fighting.

Now, since you're a Miracle Kid your white blood will win and will kill all the buggies. But here's the deal, when they fight they make your intestines get all puffy and swollen, because your intestines don't like all that fighting in them. With everyone knocking each other around and hitting the walls of your intestines, your intestines are getting hurt and swollen. So your intestines tell your body to hurry up and win and stop the fighting. So, your body gets really, really, hot.

So, you know how daddy doesn't like the heat? It makes him cranky and uncomfortable? Now, if it was mommy fighting, I would love the heat! But the buggies are like daddy—they don't like the heat. So your body thinks, "If I get it hot enough the buggies will stop fighting and the white blood will win!!!" The problem is the white blood is getting hot too!! And they are getting tired from the heat and can't fight as much. They are sweating, Em!! So, if you take your Tylenol, your body will cool off and your white blood won't be so hot, and it will kick the buggy's butt! But they need YOU to help them by taking the Tylenol!

Stupid Tumor doesn't want you to take it! Stupid Tumor wants your white blood to be hot so the buggies will win!!! You can do it Em…(I take her hand and look her square in the eye.) Mommy always tells you the truth, right? I'm telling you, you can do this. I know it will hurt, and I know you can do it anyway. I know you are the strongest kid I know. I know you are stronger than your tumor. I know you can do it."

We order up two Tylenols including a backup in case she spits them out; I'm prepared…thinking ahead.

#1 goes in.

#1 gets spit out.

No worries. Remember, I have a back up.

#2 goes in.

#2 gets spit out.

I have the most strong-willed child on the planet. So much for the backup.

"Em, you are wasting meds! You can't spit them out. There won't be enough for the other kids." She looks at me, narrows her defiant gray/green eyes, her one little naked shoulder shrugs up at me, and she arches one hairless eyebrow at me as if to say, "So what?"

We order two more.

"Em that's not your best. I need you to do your best…do you hear that? Do you? It's Stupid Tumor! He's having a party in Pathology! You spit them out! All the tumors are high fiving! They're saying, "We knew she couldn't do it! Ha ha! She can't! She can't!

Come on Em—I know you can. That wasn't your best. No, I'm not going to rub your feet. You didn't do your best. I know you can. Remember our deal? I take care of you. You do your best."

Fifteen minutes pass waiting for the new meds to come up.

#3 goes in.

2/3 gets spit out.

1/3 is in! Small victory!

She screams. Her mouth is burning. I give her water.

Give me #4—,the RN is surprised at my persistence. "She can do it," I say. "I know she can. Come on Em. I need your best."

#4 goes in.

1/3 gets spit out.

"We're going to keep doing it Em until you take it, because I know you can."

The rest goes in. She swallows!

Victory!

"Do you hear that Em? Do you hear that? You don't? It sounds like…"No!!! No!!! She did it!!! She did it!!!" Stupid Tumor is screaming!! The other tumors know you took it!! "Stupid Tumor we TOLD you not to mess with a Miracle Kid!" Em, you did it! You did it! I knew you could! You did your BEST!!! I know it was hard. I know it hurt. You can do anything, Em! You ARE a Miracle Kid!! I am so proud of you because you did your best!!! The white blood is saying, "Yayaya she did it! Take THAT buggies, we're kicking your butt!"

Em looks at me. She smiles through her blood-stained lips. Her sheet wiggles. She's shakin' her booty at Stupid Tumor. She's a fighter. She's victorious. She's my Miracle Kid.

Take that, Stupid Tumor.

i can't hear you. weLL, now neither can eM

As part of her "work up" to get ready to go into BMT., Emily had to go through a number of different tests. First up, she had her first dentist visit. Poor kid, after all she had been through, she was scared to go to the dentist. It took half an hour for the transport people to figure out how to get one kid, one wagon, one "pole" with a feeding tube and fluids, a mom, a gorilla and pig (they were the stuffed animals who made the "cut" this morning and got to go on a trip to the

super cool, fun dentist) into a van to get her to the dentist.

When we got into the room, we decided the X-ray machine looked like an ostrich head. I was, of course, jealous it "kissed" her on her nose, chin, and cheek and didn't kiss me! "No fair!" I said. I told her there was no way she could bite on the black cookie (X-ray film) and hold it in her mouth. I was sure she couldn't. She grinned and held her bite. Then she laughed and laughed that she knew she could do it! We counted gorilla's teeth. He only had 15, she had 20. Hers were even, his weren't…even funnier.

Then they told us she brushes better than some 7-year-olds they've seen. (Insert mom pride here!) I have to say it was my first time sitting as the parent watching her brush her teeth while the dentist watched her, so I was thinking…"Come on, do it right kid! Show them I'm a good parent and that I've taught you to brush your teeth the right way." Phew! I passed.

EKG & Echocardiograms…. results are in…they are good!

Hearing test. First test comes back and her results are off from what they were in December. Okay, let's do more testing. Second test. Her ear is healthy, so it's not from the Corona virus she has. (Yes, it's actually called Corona virus…basically a cold.) Third test. Emily sits in the chair. Little earphones on her tiny ears. She has to place a toy into a box every time she hears the "bird" chirp in her ear. I see the doctor writing notes. I don't know what they mean, however I'm thinking it's not good. Not sure why, I mean, maybe those circles are good circles?

Then they put the little mini ear phone on her ear bone. I hear the high "beep" tone. I hear it again. And then a third time. Each time louder. Em sits there holding the block waiting to hear the beep. I turn her feeding tube off. It must be that crunch crunch sound it makes as it turns that's interfering with her being able to hear that beep.

Again, I hear the beep. I hear it a little louder. A little louder. On the fourth beep, Em puts the block in the box. She doesn't know she didn't hear the first three. It's all a game to her. I put my hand to my mouth. I'm big into energy. I don't want my sudden fear to "reach" her.

After the "game" is over, I look at the doctor. I'm holding back tears. She confirms. Emily has suffered "moderate" hearing loss. It's from her two rounds of that awful Cisplatin chemotherapy. It's known for hearing loss.

Okay, I think, so she can't hear a high pitch. No biggie right. Then the doctor continues. It could get worse.

They don't know if it will, they can't stop it if it does, and they can't reverse this damage that is now permanent. Okay, I think, well it won't get worse. Like everything else, I'll just make up my mind it won't. I'm not crying. Em can tell I'm rattled. She keeps fussing and won't sit still. She's picking up on my energy. She'll need two hearing aids. One in each ear. "What?!?!? I'm sorry, I must have the hearing problem now. What did you just say? How can this be? If we didn't even know she had hearing loss until your stupid little birdie beeping test then why would she need a hearing aid? Obviously, it's not affecting her day to day!" Well, I learn, actually it is. She hears fish…but only hears the "ish." It's only because she used to hear the "F" that her brain fills in the blank. She is missing sounds and not realizing it. Hearing aids will help her fill in those gaps. I hate cancer.

Well, it can't be that bad. I mean, I've seen the commercials and hearing aids are like little tiny nothings now… no one will see them. Wrong. Kids her age need the big ones that hook behind their ears. She won't be able to get a small in-the-ear kind until she's 15 or so. "Seriously? Isn't there a surgery or something they can do to fix these little 'inner ear hairs?' I mean it's 2010!!!"

Nope. Science is working on it. Nothing yet. Maybe in the future. Right now she is stuck with ear jewelry.

Em is now getting upset because she doesn't understand what we are talking about. "Tell me!" she cries. She always says this to me when she knows we're talking about treatment for her. How do I explain to her she can't hear things she thinks she can? After all, I just praised her at how fabulous she did at her "beeping" game. I hate cancer.

Here's a Peek into How it Went:

The doctor shows her a picture of an ear…it shows the inner ear. I explain that she has little "hairs" in her ears that help her hear. I wiggle my fingers to demonstrate the little hairs. I say they hear high beeps [said in a high voice]. And they hear low beeps [said in a low voice]. High beeps [high voice] low beeps [low voice].

I ask her, "So when we take our GCSF (the white blood stimulator that we inject into her leg after chemo) what does it do?" She knows this answer. "Wake up!!" she yells…that's right… it goes though her body and tells her white blood to WAKE UP!

"Well," I explain, "your little ear hairs have gotten tired from the chemo. It made them {insert yawn}

fall asleep" {stop wiggling fingers to show they are sleeping}. So we need to wake them up because they can't hear the high beeps! So we get ear jewelry that you wear on your ears, and it goes into your ear and says "WAKE UP!" {Lift fingers to show hair is now awake}. "So it goes asleep {drop fingers} and it wakes up" {lift fingers}. This makes sense to her, but I'm not fully convinced she's okay with it. I'm not. I hate cancer.

We leave the room, and I walk her down the fifteen hundred mile walk back to her room. Holding back tears. I don't want to see her little bald head touting two large hearing aids. I don't want her to have a visible reminder every day of her life about cancer. I want to complete her treatment, be done, and ten years from now think, that was a lifetime ago. Not be reminded regularly that I hate cancer. I don't want people to look at her. My thoughts rush to her in school. I don't want kids to make fun of her. I don't want her to be dateless. I don't want her to be self-conscious. To think she is anything less than perfect. I am keenly aware that I seem most upset about "what other people will think." This is odd for me. I don't usually care what other people think. She doesn't ever want to grow her hair back and has told me on more than one occasion if it grows back that she is cutting it off. So maybe she won't care she has hearing aids. I do. I wonder what other long-term side effects she will have. Will I look back at these effects and wonder if the cure will be worth the quality of life she will have? Or will these "effects" be such a part of her she won't know any different kind of "quality of life." After all, she asked the emergency room nurse for her Oxycodone and Atavan upon admittance. She knows the words broviac, CAT scan, catheter, chest tube, tumor, B.M.T., and biopsy. Maybe her world is so different already that a hearing aid or two will be nothing.

I get back to the seventh floor. The kid in the room next to Emily is dying. The Colors of Life were just taped to their door. It's from the chaplain's bereavement services.

Suddenly, a hearing aid doesn't seem so bad. I think they even come in some cool colors now.

Rudolph Wears a Pirates Hat

A few months after Emily's cancer treatment was almost over, we noticed a huge mole growing on the inside of her left leg. Of course any mom would be nervous about a strange growth on their child's leg, but as a cancer mom "nervous" takes on a whole new meaning. The paralyzing fear that it could be cancer-related no doubt crossed my mind more than once. Her oncologist gave me a referral and sent us to the dermatology wing of the hospital.

After an exam, the dermatologist determined it was not a cancerous mole (sigh of relief). However, it was pretty ugly and would continue to grow. So yes, it needed to be removed and a plastic surgeon would do the procedure. I wasn't too pleased with this. After all, who was this unknown plastic surgeon? Didn't they realize only my miracle surgeon Dr. Bruny was allowed to operate on my Miracle Kid? Apparently not. Well, I rationalized, it was just a mole so we would get through it. Now I had to figure out how to make a mole fun.

Here's a peek into how it went:

As we were sitting in the doctor's office looking at this ugly red mole I looked over at Emily and asked, "So what do you think its name is?"

After quickly looking it over, she decided his name was, "Rudolph." Then came the flood of questions. "What is it mom? Why is there on my leg? What does it do?"

I had no scientific answers, so I did what I always did when I got caught having to explain unknown medical situations: I made it fun. Thinking on my feet, I quickly responded that her body knew Tumor was in Pathology getting pokes and chops and tormented all day, every day. But her body was worried that Tumor might try to sneak out. After all, I reasoned, he was a sneaky tumor because he had snuck into her body in the first place! Well, I continued, her body had done everything it could to make sure Tumor couldn't get back into her. I began to list all the fun things she had done: Karate Fox Chemo, Boot Camp for her Stem Cells, Radiation to put sun in her so Tumor couldn't hide, etc. But her body didn't want Tumor getting out of Pathology, and so her body (cells) had gotten together and had grown Rudolph. Her Doctor would take him off and send him to Pathology too. Rudolph would guard the door and make sure Tumor couldn't get out.

Well, Emily loved the idea that Rudolph was her own personal bodyguard. "What do you think Rudolph will need to guard Stupid Tumor?" I asked her. She decided he needed a pirate's sword and a pirate's hat. I thought that was a pretty good idea,

so we talked about Rudolph and how he would be taken to Pathology with his pirate's hat and sword.

Months later, we would still talk about how every time Stupid Tumor even looked at the exit door there was Rudolph ready to cut him up, poke him, and push him back into his little tumor box. We would talk about how Rudolph loves his job guarding Stupid Tumor, and there is no way Tumor could every get out. I reminded her that only a Miracle Kid would have her own private bodyguard.

*It's important to note I have never been to or seen a pathology lab. I actually have no idea what they really do with the tumor once it's removed. Emily is enrolled in a number of national studies, so I am assuming at least part of her tumor was or is being studied. However, I sincerely doubt the tumor is kept in a box. And that's my point. Emily was 4 at this time. She had no more understanding of a pathology department than I did at 34. So whatever I could imagine up in my mind became reality for both of us. A mole guarding a tumor is crazy silly, but it worked.

HeaRiNG HelPeRS

Describing why Emily needed to wear hearing aids was one thing. Actually getting her to wear them was something different.

I tried all different names besides calling them hearing aids. First I called them "ear jewelry," but as her audiologist pointed out that was not the best term because jewelry is something you wear at your discretion. Sometimes you want to wear jewelry, and sometimes you don't. It made it too much of an option to not wear her hearing aids, so in the end I decided to call them "Hearing Helpers." This also proved valuable down the road when Emily started school, because when other kids would ask, "Hey what are those things in your ear?" I could simply say, "Those are her Hearing Helpers, they help her hear," which made a lot of sense to kids.

When she started kindergarten, she went into school on an IEP, an Individual Education Program. It allowed her to receive services for her hearing aids, including speech therapy and hearing support. One of the services was to provide an FM system, a hearing system that basically magnifies the teacher's voice. Emily wears what we call a little "boot" on her hearing aid, which then hooks into a microphone that the teacher wears like a necklace. So, no matter where she is teaching in the room, it sounds like she is within three feet of Emily's ear. It makes a huge difference, especially when it comes to background noise, which as you can imagine, in a kindergarten, or a first grade or second grade, classroom it can get a little noisy.

When Emily first had her "boots" put on and the FM system set up, a lot of the kids were naturally curious to know what it was all about. So after running it by me, the teachers decided to have her explain to her peers what her hearing aids did. The plan was to bring her up to the front of the kindergarten room and share how her hearing aids worked.

Later, I received a call from her hearing support teacher who was quite distraught. Apparently, while Emily was in the front of the room, the teacher asked her to share why she wore hearing aids. Instead of answering the way her teacher anticipated (I'm thinking she expected her to say, "They help me hear,") my 5-year-old answered confidently, "Because I had cancer."

I guess using the C word, even in kindergarten, makes other people uncomfortable. I wasn't uncomfortable. Emily wasn't uncomfortable. That truly is why she wears hearing aids, and it really didn't matter to me what Emily wanted to share with the class. I'm glad that Emily can use the word "cancer" without any negative connotation. She had cancer the same as if somebody had the chickenpox, or the flu, or tonsillitis.

Putting her hearing aids in on her own was something that took a while for her to learn. Suspiciously enough, I found out from the kindergarten specialist that she was quite efficient at being able to put her hearing aids in and to take them out at school. However, at home it proved a different story. She always wanted me to put them in and "couldn't" do it herself. Hmm.... I also found it challenging how to teach someone else how to put her hearing aids in for her, particularly when she was only 4 and 5 years old.

To make it easier to teach other people, and of course to make it fun, we developed a little song.

We put the hearing aid in on it's side and we would sing:

> You hook and you twist
>
> and it goes like this.
>
> Then you wrap, you wrap,
>
> you wrap around the back.

The "hook" was sticking the ear mold part of the hearing aid in the ear. The "twist" was twisting the ear mold into place and the "wrap" was putting the hearing aid body itself behind her ear.

We loved to sing the hook and twist, and we taught it to other family members in case they forget how to put Emily's hearing aids in. They'd remember when she'd sing with them, "You hook and you twist and it goes like this. Then you wrap, you wrap, you wrap around the back." It's funny how this little song became so "normal" to us!

Strep...it's fun

Making medical fun goes beyond life-threatening, critical illnesses. Just to give you an example: after Emily was off treatment, she got sick and I had to take her to a pediatrician appointment. She had been running a fever and had a sore throat. Just normal kid first-grade sickness. How great to be able to take care of a sick kid when it doesn't involve a hospital or emergency room visit. The pediatrician opted to do a flu test and a strep test because she was running such a high fever. No kid, or adult for that matter, likes a flu or a strep test where you end up gagging.

Here's all the "fun" we (or should I say she) had. First, she got to pee on my hand. They wanted a urine test just to make sure she didn't have a urinary tract infection, and it's always more fun to pee when you know mom's hand is getting peed on too. So that started it. Then to do the flu test, she had to blow boogers out of her nose so they could catch them on a Q-Tip. Well it is more fun to blow boogers into your mom's hand than it is to do anything else. So she got to blow boogers onto my hand, which caused me to make gross, disgusting, barfing faces and noises. Emily thought this was hysterical.

Afterwards, we had to wait for the results of her rapid strep test. Sitting in the doctor's office bored, Emily started asking lots of questions: "What is a strep test? How does it work? What does it do?" Put on the spot, I had to think of a way to explain the science of strep and a Petri dish in 6-year-old terminology.

Here's a peek into how it went:

Thinking fast (and thinking FUN), I explained that the doctor takes these little round plastic dishes called Petri dishes, and inside it's kind of like Disneyland for germs. There are roller coasters, rides, games, and a pool, and your test is going to trick those buggies!

Here's how: "Those buggies are going to jump out of your nose or out of your throat, out of your spit, and out of your boogers. We're going to put your boogers inside that dish that has a Disneyland for germs. Those little buggies are hiding in your boogers, but when they get into the Petri dish and they see how cool Disneyland is, they're going to want to come out

of the boogers and go on the roller coasters, and go play in the pool, and go check it all out. And that's when we trick them! If they come out of those boogers and they start playing on the roller coaster, we'll know that they were hiding there in your boogers! Once we know they're there, then the doctor can give you medicine to kill them all over your body. It's the same thing with your strep test. Your little buggies are hiding in your spit. We're going to put them in the Petri dish, and those little buggies are going to want to crawl out of your spit and go play so we can find them! We're very tricky. You are very tricky. Those buggies think they can hide in your boogers and spit, but we're going to find them!"

I try to take a concept that might be really difficult for a child to understand and explain it in a way that is fun. At the same time, what kid doesn't want to trick all of her germs and bugs that are making her feel sick, and trap them, and kill them, be the winner, and be victorious? So, even with small medical procedures it's a great way to start thinking, "How can I explain this to a child that makes sense, that doesn't feel scary, and that doesn't feel threatening." I just use my imagination and picture myself like a child. Confession time! A lot of times the ideas I came up with were simply because I really didn't know either! I didn't know the medical terminology. I didn't know exactly how that Petri dish worked, but it made sense to me and sounded fun. My job has never been to be a medical guru; it's always been to keep my kid smiling.

Fun Factor

Tips for thinking on your feet:

Use your senses.
* What does it look like?
* What does it feel like?
* Does it smell?
* Does it make a sound?
* Does it have a taste?

What color is it?
* When you think of that color, what is the first thing that pops into your head?
* What are 3 things associated with that color?

Think like a kid.
* If you were 3 years old, how would you describe this?
* If you had to draw a picture of it, what would you draw?

Stumped?
* Ask your Miracle Kid the same questions! Ask them to use their five senses!

Still stumped?
* Ask the doctor or medical professional if they can give you an analogy, something to help you understand better.

People are Staring at the Tube in your Nose

I found it fascinating to watch how adults would react to Emily's differences versus how children did. Remember, she had a nose tube for most of her treatment. (Pretty common in the Club Cancer). A long yellow tube that stuck out of her nose was taped across her cheek onto her face and hung down. Her feeding tube was what allowed us to "hook" into her food at night, especially when she couldn't eat. I found it fascinating that for a long time, even though she was completely bald, the kids never seemed to notice her alien-like head. They were, however, fascinated by this feeding tube that sadly remained up her nose up until the very end of treatment. So, even after she was going home between her bio-therapies, she still had this yellow tube stuck in her nose.

Kids would point and stare in wonder, but of course adults would take one glance at her bald head and would know exactly why she had a feeding tube. They would get uncomfortable, glance away, and tell their kids quietly, "Stop doing that. Don't look. That's not nice."

I know they had the best intentions. I know it's hard to know how each individual family is going to react to another child or adult staring. Emily and I, we choose to embrace the stares. It wasn't that they were being rude or hurtful; kids are just naturally curious. Why did this kid have a long yellow tube sticking out of her nose?

Here's a peek into how it went:

"Is that spaghetti in her nose?" a kid might ask. (Don't you just love their innocence?)

When kids would point or stare, or I could tell they wanted to ask a question, even if the parent shooed them away, I would crouch down, look at them, and say, "Wanna know why she has a tube in her nose, huh?" They'd always look at me wide-eyed and nod their head yes!

I'd say, "Well, we put food in the tube, and she eats through her nose. It helps her eat. Pretty cool, huh?" Every single kid nodded their head in agreement. It was pretty cool that you could eat through your nose. I think it's all about how you handle it. It wasn't scary. It wasn't gross. Kids love gross stuff. They like to pull boogers out of their noses and eat them or stick string down their nose to see if it comes out their mouth. The idea that Emily could put food down her nose and eat, well that was pretty cool. I would grin, Emily would grin, and they would grin. Then, of course, their parents would always look super relieved.

Only when Emily started pre-school did we have a hard time with how she looked. She had just finished treatment and her hair was starting to grow back in. It was super short and looked like she had a military buzz cut. In all honesty she did look a little like a boy. Even though I dressed her in lots of pink and purple, people would still refer to her as "He." Some kids in the preschool class would even ask her if she was a boy or a girl. Fortunately, hair grows fast and it was only for a very short period of time. Since she refused to wear headbands, scarves, or anything else that would make her look like a girl, she looked more like a boy then she probably wanted. I simply explained to her that kids just didn't know. It wasn't to be mean, they weren't making fun, they just didn't know because normally girls have long hair and normally boys have short hair.

We talked about how even "normal" wasn't true for everyone, pointing out the girls we knew who had short hair and the boys we knew who had long hair. I only remember a handful of incidents with Emily being upset because kids couldn't tell she was a boy or a girl, but if you asked her today I doubt she would even remember. How grateful I am my memory is better than hers.

It's always best, if you have a chance, to prepare in advance on how you want to respond to a situation—unlike the situations described before when you aren't prepared and are just thrown into the circus! One issue the majority of Miracle Kids will have to deal with is their appearance. Bald heads, feeding tubes, chemo bags, and masks stand out. Even more so for anyone dealing with an amputation, disfigurement, or more permanent issues. Deciding together ahead of time how you want to handle the unusual stares, points, and questions can empower both you and your child to respond instead of react.

Fun Factor

What are some things people might notice about your child that look "different"?

_____

_____

_____

_____

_____

_____

_____

If your child is old enough, decide together how you want to respond. (Give them control). Explain that people are curious, not mean, but they may never have seen a Miracle Kid in person before!

For each thing, decide ahead of time how you want to respond to curious looks or questions:

Someone might be curious about:	If it's an adult, here's how I'll choose to respond.	If it's a child, here's how I'll choose to respond.

A Peek Into Our World—I Think I Have a Child With Special Needs

I say "I think" because I don't want to say it at all. I don't want a child with special needs. I want a child who had cancer, kicked its butt, and now is "normal."

Yesterday, Emily came with me to the post office. I walked behind her. All arms and legs, 4-years-old, just 33 pounds and super tall. (So far radiation has NOT stunted any growth!) She is lanky and skinny. She bounded in with a nose tube hanging out of the right side of her face, which is two-thirds covered by her B.M.T. mask that is her shield against the world of germs. Her right arm is wrapped in CoBand, tucking in the two new Pic IV lines that will stay there until December. Her sneakers are bursting at the sides from her new orthotics that come up around her ankles, and her two new hearing aids are on either side of her head.

The orthotics have animal prints on them. I tried to make it fun that she was stepping on a monkey with each step she took. So, between the jungle print orthotics, the hot pink and orange "ear jewelry," (her choice of colors), her neon pink CoBand wrapped around her arm, and her bright turquoise mask, the kid is quite a fashion statement. As I watched her in that moment it was the first time I saw her as a kid with special needs. All those flashing colors proclaiming to the world....I am not "normal." I have...ugh my stomach turns as I type this..."disabilities." It was almost as if for the first time I saw her as other people see her.

It's strange that in almost nine months I have never seen her as a "special needs" kid. Even though her bedroom looks like a medical storage room...bins of syringes, Tagaderm tape, a huge "Tree" pole for her feeding pump, backpacks and pumps for her TPN, bottles of saline, heparin, sterile water, and more creams, lotions, and drugs than a pharmacy. Still, it's just her room. She's just my kid. It's just part of cancer. And it's not forever.

Today, forever hit. Even when cancer is over, the effects are not. "Long-term side effects." It's something you don't hear much about while you're going through treatment. When I ask about them, I get vague generalities. Partly because no one knows. (I mean really, this is the first generation of kids who live through her type of cancer to have long-term side effects.) Everyone is all too aware of the reality, that she may not be around to have long term-side effects. They think why worry about that yet? Let's hope she has long-term side effects that we'll have to deal with. This seems to be the general consensus. Any side effects are worth survival. Long-Term Effects = Life = Victory.

Of all the things this kid has gone through, of all the "badges of courage" she has (2 chest tube scars, the "diamond cut" across her abdomen, the small pencil-eraser-shaped scars that cover her chest from various stitches, lung surgery, and biopsies), her hearing aids bother me the most. Maybe it's because I can't put a shirt over them. Maybe it's because without hair, their bright neon colors scream, "I CAN'T HEAR!" Maybe it's because they remind me every time I look at her that I hate cancer. Maybe it's because I don't want her to have long-term side effects. After all, she's my Miracle Kid. Miracle Kids don't have long-term side effects. Or maybe that's what being a Miracle Kid means. You get to have long-term side effects because you lived. You survived. You were victorious.

I wonder how many people were looking at her as she bounced her way into the post office totally oblivious that she is different. That she is now a "special needs" kid.

We just got her "ear jewelry" this morning.* I have to say at least they really do look like "jewelry." We've gotten so used to calling it ear jewelry, that when the audiologist handed her a book about an elephant and his hearing aids the words "hearing aids" threw me off. Wait. I thought we were getting ear jewelry? Hearing aids just do not sound as fun or as cool. Fortunately she is 4, so hot pink and orange ear jewelry is cool.

Then, Stephanie came in the room. She works at the hospital in the audiology department and talks to all the families when they come in to actually get their hearing aids. I never really caught what her actual job was. Maybe hospital Angel?

She has a hearing aid in one ear. In the other, a Cochlear implant. You can't see them. Her chin-length bob covers them. Other than her speech, she "looks" normal. She's pretty. Very pretty. I'm sitting there as she is talking to me thinking, "Wow, she seems so normal." With a flash of guilt I think, "Why would I think someone hard of hearing is not normal?" I have no idea. I have to admit that I guess subconsciously I do. I must if I was surprised she was normal. She has a wedding ring on. Someone married this woman! I wonder what her husband is like. Does he care his wife is....

*ok wait, I don't even know the politically correct term....Hard of hearing? Hearing disabled? Hearing impaired? Part way deaf!?? I guess I should find out because now it describes my daughter... I decide I'll Google it.

I am shocked by my ignorance. I am relieved she is married. Someone wanted to marry her. Maybe someone will still want to marry Emily even if she can't hear. Here is this beautiful, well dressed, married, well spoken, put together woman, and she has a hearing aid! Doesn't seem to affect her much. She pops it and out and shows Emily. Like it is an earring. I wanted to ask her if she went to her prom. I mean, getting married is one thing...by the time you get married I would hope people don't care about a little thing like a hearing aid. But the prom? Will Em be the 6-foot 3-inch dateless deaf girl who needs to take her cousin to the prom? Will she need to wear orthotics with her flat shoes because she'll be too tall to wear heels? Will we have to have the hair dresser try to style her hair to cover her hearing aids and have to find a dress that covers the blue veins that come up her chest to her left arm because of a clot her broviac left? I have this horrible mental picture of a prom photo of Emily. The only thing worse is that for some reason I also picture her in head gear and a mouth full of metal.

*When Em first got her hearing aids we called them "ear jewelry" to make it sound fun. In retrospect, that wasn't a great idea because jewelry is an optional accessory. Later we changed it to "hearing helpers" because wearing them wasn't optional.

I am a terrible person.
My child has fought for nine months to kick cancer's butt.
She has endured weeks of NPO (nothing by mouth) crying that she was hungry.

She has endured months of having a chest tube tying her to a bed making her scared to take a step.

She has endured physical therapy, occupational therapy, and breathing therapy.

She has endured an eight-hour surgery that resulted in a picture from her surgeon that was so disgusting and gory it didn't even look like a person. The only give-a-way was the belly button at the bottom of the picture reminding you this was her stomach!

She has endured internal mucositis sores running from her mouth to her butt that were so painful she was on a narcotic drip.

She has endured cyclical vomiting—puking every 15 minutes for 10 days and getting acid burns on her chin from the vomit.

She has endured 104.5 fevers, being packed down with ice, ER admissions, twice daily injections into her skinny little legs, and dressing changes all over.

She has endured a week of bio therapy with blood pressures 50/20 in the PICU (Pediatric Intensive Care Unit).

And what I do care about?

Getting her a prom date.

Really, I am sure my thoughts alone are offensive to every special needs family and child out there. Am I that vain? I did pray when she was in my belly that she would be pretty. I will defend myself by quoting a new study that shows pretty people actually make more money than non-attractive people.

As I watch her, I realize she is not normal. She is beautiful. She is funny. Everyone in the hospital who meets her loves this kid. She has a reputation. She is more self assured than any 4-year-old should ever have to be, and she is a child with special needs.

Maybe, just maybe, somehow her special needs reflect on me and threaten me since, after all, I seem to be the only one with the issue about her ear jewelry. She does not seem to care. I tried to make it fun. I told her I was jealous, I wanted ear jewelry. I asked to borrow them. Asked if I could get a matching pair. She told me no. I begged the audiologist. She told me no. I told her C & A (the two other kids with the same Neuroblastoma and same therapy) didn't get ear jewelry. It must just be for Miracle Kids but that she should not tell them that because they would be jealous. I dramatically gagged and told her the longer she wears them the more ear wax I would have to clean off and that I couldn't handle the gross stuff like she could. She loved it and said she would wear them all the time. This kid loves to gross me out. Other than trying to get used to how they feel, she doesn't seem to care at all that her ear jewelry makes her different. She does double check to make sure I took the orange "necklace" with us because she wants to wear that jewelry too. (It's a string that hooks to the back of the hearing aids and clips to the back of her shirt so they don't fall off or get lost. They are really more for babies, but Emily loves jewelry, and to her it's just another "accessory.") I mean really, this is the same kid who is begging me to shave her head now that her hair is growing back in, and she doesn't want to have to wash it. Having hot pink and orange in her ears is nothing. The mask will come off next week. The nose tube isn't permanent. The Pic Line is there until December. And even her broviac will eventually come out. Her hair will grow in and cover her hearing aids, and in the winter she'll wear boots and no one will see her orthotics. All the "externals" will change. She will look "normal." Although, I'm not sure what that means any more.

She was so angry the other day playing outside with the neighborhood girls. She couldn't keep up with them on their bikes. She was frustrated that her legs tire more easily. She started crying. I held her and cried with her because she wasn't as "strong" as they were. My kid, who is kicking cancer's butt. Cancer that kills even the toughest of men, that stumps even the smartest of scientists to find a cure. Cancer that strikes fear in the hearts of most grownups just upon its utterance. That cancer. She is kicking its butt. She is waging war on "Stupid Tumor." She reminds Stupid Tumor daily that she hates him. She takes her meds even when she doesn't want to and reminds Stupid Tumor he is staying in Pathology. She tells Stupid Tumor he has no friends. And she asks me regularly if I also hate Stupid Tumor, I do. She looked at me the other day and said, "Mommy, my tumor's still that word that you won't let me say." She has a personal vendetta against Stupid Tumor. It's her or him, and she's decided she's winning. I think, bikes or not, she is the strongest kid I know. She asked me at the clinic last week if I thought A & C were strong too. I told her any kid that kicks cancer's butt is strong. These kids are little warriors, and they don't even know it.

I take a deep breath. She's in bed, and the hearing aids are sitting in their "jewelry box" on her night stand. Her pump is running her TPN, her feedbag is running her formula feeds, and she is curled up next to me in her bed. I kiss her fuzzy head. I miss that bald head. Time marches on. Life will go on. One day her room will be "normal" and won't have all these supplies, and I won't need to bring out a new garbage bag each night full of medical trash just from trying to get her ready for bed. Like all "normal" kids, she will start school, have homework, go to sleepovers, and, hopefully, have a prom date. Life will be "normal." Our days will be "normal." And bedtime routines will be "normal."

But Em....

she will not...

she will still be...special.

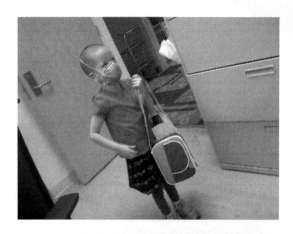

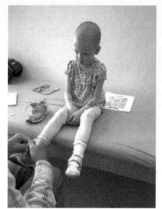

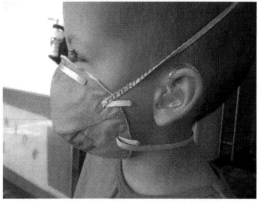

The first day Em got her hearing aids and the first time she got her orthotics.

You've Been taking Care of Your Miracle Kid, But Have You Been taking Care of You?

My Secrets to Sanity

Up to 30% of fathers and 40% of mothers may exhibit moderate to severe symptoms of post-traumatic stress (PTS) [after a childhood cancer diagnosis] ~ cancernetwork.com.

Create a Grateful Journal

If you only utilize one tool from this book, I hope this is it. This is the one thing that made the biggest difference for me, and I believe it has the power to change your life if you let it. Yup, it's that big. Let me paint you the picture of what my life was like BC and then maybe you'll understand why this one tool is so powerful. When Emily was diagnosed, it was just nine short months after my divorce. The year prior, I had endured one of the most difficult things I have ever gone through (and yes, I say this as the mom of a Miracle Kid). I went through a domestic violence divorce. It was one of the scariest times of my life. Prayers were interwoven with weeping, pleading, begging, and bargaining. Months of court battles left me emotionally, physically, and financially exhausted. I thought I had hit rock bottom.

It turns out I was just sitting on a trap door and there was much further to fall. Fast forward, and I find myself a single mother of a child with a childhood cancer diagnosis. Literally, in the emergency room, I was informed that my ex-husband's lawyer

> " Always laugh when you can. It is good medicine.
>
> Lord Byron "

was contacting the hospital to have me removed the next morning so he could exercise his parenting time. A friend drove my mother two hours roundtrip to get my court paperwork so I could show the hospital I was the only one with medical decision making ability and that I had a restraining order. Childhood cancer is a living nightmare. When you add domestic violence on top of it, it's like a nightmare in hell. Then, three days later I received a phone call that the owner of the company I had recently signed onto to be a spokeswoman for had just unexpectedly passed away and everything (including my paycheck) was on hold…indefinitely. And finally, the guy I had just started dating politely removed himself from my current crisis.

As you can imagine, all I could focus on was what was falling apart around me. I remember crying to God about how I thought life was bad from my divorce but that I would take back that life in a minute. Childhood cancer was too much. I also knew from all my years immersed in the personal development world that what you focus on gets bigger. I knew I needed to change my focus…fast. One night sitting on the oncology floor, watching my Miracle Baby sleep, I logged into Facebook

and started the one thing that changed everything: my grateful journal. Here's a peek into that first entry:
Written January 14, 2010 at 9:36 p.m.
~ Less than 8 weeks after diagnosis

"So, I'm realizing how ungrateful I have been. These last two years, I have been feeling sorry for myself. Those of you who know me well will probably agree that while I may have earned a certain amount of self pity time I have also failed to see the blessings I did and do have. It's strange how my child has cancer, yet my body is the one that's changing. My eyes see differently, my heart beats softer, my body moves slower, and my mind is slowly being taken over by my right brain (who, up until now, lefty and I successfully managed to squash anytime she tried to raise her vulnerable voice) so to be accountable (oh, Facebook, you have so many uses), I'm listing my gratefulness here:
Today I'm grateful for:
My mom being able to stay with Em at the hospital when I have to leave.
My cousin being able to stay with my mom.

And so on.

That first night, I listed 18 things I was grateful for. Yes 18! The second night I listed 19 things. Just a couple of weeks later on February 5th I listed 36 things! By April 5th I wrote the words: "Life is Good," the first time in my life I could claim those words. My daughter still had cancer. I still didn't know if she would live, but I still could say life was good. If that's not powerful, I'm not sure what is!

Put it into Practice:

- Create your own Grateful Journal. You can use a laptop or a notebook.
- Your notebook doesn't need to be anything fancy, but I have found having a beautiful book to write in makes me want to pick it up!
- Commit to write in your Grateful Journal for at least 21 days straight. (It takes 21 days to create a new habit.)
- Commit to listing a minimum of 5 things each night. Force yourself to dig deeper and find more things to be grateful for.
- Try to not repeat the same 5 things each day. For example, if you have 4 kids and a spouse, that could be your same 5 over and over! That defeats the purpose! The reason we are creating a Grateful Journal is to force us to recognize and acknowledge the good things around us and the blessings we are missing.
- Don't feel pressure to think of "big" things to be grateful for. Sometimes it's the small things that are the biggest gratitude givers.

tips to Prompt your Gratitude:

Who are you grateful for?

- Family
- Parents
- Friends
- Co-Workers
- Neighbors

Real Life Example from my GJ (Grateful Journal): *"For Bethany and John (again) who came and brought lots of food but also four shoulders for leaning on and helping me sort through all my feelings."*

What are you grateful for?

- Home
- YOUR health
- Job
- Car (I saw many families waiting outside for the bus they took back and forth to the hospital.)

Real Life Example from my GJ: *"That we have more than one puke bucket in the room."*

Big wins you can be grateful for:

- A test that comes back with great results.
- Getting through a test/scan/lab work/ round of chemo or radiation.
- A milestone checked off your goal poster.

- Getting discharged from the hospital for some time at home.

Real Life Example from my GJ: *"For our first "tree free!" ride in the wagon…we are off TPN, no chest tube, and down to just 1 IV antibiotic (all other meds are by mouth)…so the only thing "attached" to Em is her feeding tube in her nose…Dr Ben wheeled and dealed with her that she could get one hour free detached from the tube to "cruise" downstairs…in exchange for drinking a non-fat nutritional shake."*

Small wins you can be grateful for:

- How are your child's blood counts? Did they get better at all today?
- Lowering of any medication doses.
- Being off precautions.
- A lowered fever.
- A new medication that your child didn't experience side effects of.
- Getting through PT, OT, or another therapy today.
- Sometimes something as small as having your child get up to brush their teeth, take a bath, or use the bathroom can be a win!

Real Life Example from my GJ: *"That Em is down to puking less than 5 times a day now."*

Things your child does or says that you are grateful for:

- What made them smile?

- What was something fun you did today?
- Did they say something that made you laugh?

Real Life Example from my GJ: *"For walking into the playroom where Em was with Aunt Chrissy. Em said,"I have a surprise for you so close your eyes," which I trustingly did…until I was shot in the pants with a syringe full of water…to which she shrieked with laughter."*

Big Picture things to be grateful for:

- The country you live in.
- The hospital at which your child is receiving treatment.
- The doctors, nurses, surgeons, and specialists who are fighting for your child's survival.
- The technology, medical advances, equipment, and drugs available to your child.
- That every day is a day for a new discovery to cure childhood cancer.

Real Life Example from my JG: *"For the person who invented feeding tubes so Emily can get the food she needs…without it I don't know how she would have pulled through."*

Small Picture things to be grateful for:

- Chocolate.
- Someone bringing a meal by.

- A chance to shower at the hospital (believe me, this small thing is a big thing!)
- A phone call from someone offering encouragement.
- A sunny day.

Real Life Example of my GJ: *"For the inventor of coffee."*

Remember what you focus on gets bigger, good or bad. It truly is a decision to choose gratefulness.

Real Life Example of my GJ: *"And sometimes when you've had a day like today… you just can be grateful today is over."*

find your faith:

Regardless of what your faith is, finding your faith and living in faith, can really make a difference. My faith gave me a sense of peace. Often, I hear people say they turned away from God during times of crisis, but for me, it was totally different. I remember when Emily was first diagnosed, people kept saying to me, "God doesn't give you what you can't handle." I would feel resentful and angry. It implied that because I was strong, that it was okay for me to be the one to have a child with cancer. While good intentioned, it almost felt mean. I told a dear friend of mine, Bethany, how I was feeling (after it was said to me the millionth time) and she shared

with me something she heard her pastor say, "God doesn't give you what you can handle. He gives you what you can't handle. That way you'll have to rely on Him." That hit me right in the heart. She was so right. I didn't feel like I could handle it. Not at all. I had to look up, because I had no place else to go. I had to get clear that God loved Emily even more than I did. And while I'm her earthly mother, He is her Father in heaven.

I remember some days when I would just sit, praying and praying and praying some more over her. Praying out a spirit of fear. Praying out a spirit of illness. Praying out a spirit of disease. Then praying to have her filled with the Holy Spirit. I can imagine for someone who doesn't have a faith in Jesus, or even in God, that would be difficult. Because when you talk about God and cancer it raises the question, why did God allow this? I never felt that God allowed this. I never felt that God gave Emily cancer. I don't even know if that was in God's plan. I believe that there is an enemy out there who wants to steal and rob us of our joy, our hope, and our faith. Why Emily had cancer, I will never know. What I did know was that God loved her.

I remember people always reminding me of Jeremiah 29:11 while I was going through my divorce. It reads, "For I know the plans I have for you," declares the LORD, "plans to prosper you and not to harm you, plans to give you hope and a future." NIV. Now in a cancer ward I would think, "How can I get peace when it gets so intensely painful and scary?" It was one day in the hospital while reading that same verse when all of a sudden I realized it wasn't God's promise just to me, it was God's promise to Emily too. God had a future for Emily planned. God had hope for Emily planned. That was His promise to her as His child. That filled me with a great sense of peace and security. I would remind myself of that verse every time fear seeped in, so I could remind myself of God's promises to Emily.

Put it into Practice:

- Does the hospital have a chapel you can use?
- Does the hospital provide daily or weekly services you can attend?

- Does the hospital have a clergy member from your particular faith you could talk to?
- Listen to faith-filled podcasts. Your church or place of worship might already put their sermons on a podcast. If not, Google or ask around for ones that might inspire you.
- Keep a Bible, Torah, Koran, or your preferred religious book in your hospital room to be able to access it when you need it.
- If you are already part of a faith community, do what you can to stay connected.
- Read inspirational and spiritual books. Ask for recommendations. Some of my favorites are:
  - *Circle Maker* by Mark Batterson
  - *Sun Stand Still* by Steven Furtick
  - *Why do Bad Things Happen to Good People* by Harold Kushner

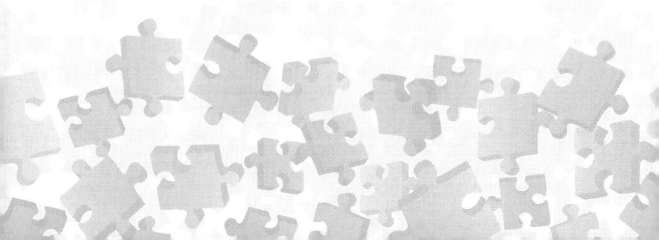

A Peek Into Our World ~ LIFE IS GOOD

Written April 5, 2010 at 1:54 a.m. ~ Five months into cancer

Tonight, Easter night, I was lying in Emily's toddler bed with her while she was falling asleep. It was dark, and we had her "relaxing" candle on. (A Melon Madness she got today when we went to get more prescriptions at Walgreens...yes you have to fight cancer even on Easter.)

As I was lying there, with her sleeping peacefully and the candle light flickering off the wall, for a moment I was at peace. A feeling of calm, fabulous, soul-singing, peace came over me.

Suddenly, I was so keenly aware that it literally had been five years since I have been able to say, "Life is good." This phrase kept playing itself over and over in my mind. "Life is good."
For the first time in my life, I now understand why people, in times of terrible grief and despair, turn their backs on God. I never understood this before. I would stand there in all my judging self-righteousness and think, why doesn't this experience turn them to God! Duh?

I knew a family who lost their grandchild to cancer. Rumor was that's what caused them to become atheists. I, of course, questioned the sincerity of their faith in the first place if they could just turn away that easily. Now, however, it's not "that easily." I have now crossed over....I'm on the "inside." I watch these kids—Logan, Zach, Zerrian, Delilah, Jonathon, Elizabeth, Amanda, April, Michael, and Emily fight for their right to life. I watch them around the 7th floor. They walk in walkers, wheel in wheel chairs or wagons, and the "cool" ones cruise on their poles, though I'm still not sure how they actually do that!

They aren't on a playground. They aren't sitting in circle time or playing flag football. They aren't wiggling in an assembly or being sent to the principal's office. They aren't worried about their clothes, boys, (or girls) or who is going out with whom (super important in 8th grade.) They aren't cramming for tests, going to the prom, or walking at graduation. No, instead they are filling their bodies with poison on a daily basis, basically killing themselves, and hoping that they won't die and that only the cancer will.

These little warriors face death at an age that seems to support belief in the devil himself. I remember learning about death through my guinea pig dying. Not because I had to ask my mom if I was going to die. The toughest question I asked my mom was what a French kiss was in 5th grade (and being grossed out by the answer).

But it's not just dying. It's dying in the most inhuman horrible way possible. It's fighting for years, puking, surgery, mucasitis (so painful these kids are put on morphine drips) pokes, tubes, meds that make you barf, and THEN you die. I now understand the neighbors. Atheism gives an answer, an answer to the "Why?!"

At the Pre-B.M.T. conference they go over each stage of treatment now that her chemo and surgery are complete. They say things like, "and kids who get to this stage..." and "then kids who get to this stage..." a subtle reminder that not all kids do. Well, Doctor, mine does. I'm not accepting anything other than 100% cure. If you told me she had a one in a million shot, I would stare you back in the face and tell you she is that one.

When my almost 4-year-old comes home and is excited because she can play in her doll house— and she wants to snuggle on the couch and "watch a little movie" and "have a relaxing night" and go to bed "with no one messing with me," —I realize these small things are what most kids do day to day and never think about, and yet for Em these are huge moments of happiness. I start to understand the atheists. How can there be a God?

And then, she is home. She is happy. It's a small victory. How can't there be? Is this small moment of happiness the "proof" there is a God, or are all the moments of fear a reminder that there's not?

Then when Emily lies on the couch reading her "David" book (about David and Goliath) and I hear her say,"But God always loves you...even if you make bad choices...God will still love you...." I'm quickly reminded that God asks me to have childlike faith. Emily faith. Faith that doesn't demand answers for cancer.

So while I am relishing my moment in a toddler bed, overwhelmed with a feeling of "peace," I am also saddened. I think about how many people really do have "good" lives and are ungrateful. I see so many get upset, angry, and riled up over the insignificant. (Don't believe me? Just read some Facebook statuses... I even dare you to read back over yours.)

I would give just about anything to be able to say that one phrase...the one that has taken root in my mind..."Life is good"

My constant prayer is that the Lord will give me peace. I can't remember the last time I felt true peace. Domestic violence turned my world upside down. Nine months later, childhood cancer spun it out of control. Peace. Elusive, evading, peace. Calmness, drama, and crisis.

So, today I'm claiming Life is good, and here's why:
I proceeded to list 29 reasons why LIFE IS GOOD!

How many can you list?

Life is Good Because:

_____

_____

_____

_____

_____

_____

_____

_____

_____

_____

_____

_____

_____

Music Moves the Soul

Want to make cancer fun? Put some music on and start dancing. There's something about music that intrinsically stirs our soul. It moves us, evokes emotion, creates us; it's amazing to me what music can do. Emily and I created different theme songs throughout her treatment. One of our favorites was Miley Cyrus' "Party in the U.S.A." which we changed to "Party in the B.M.T." We would make up silly songs and dance (or at least I would dance).

Maybe it means playing a Christian inspirational CD in your room and around you twenty-four hours a day, to fill you with a sense of peace. We loved to start our day with Mandisa's "Good Morning" to set the tone for the day.

Another song that Emily really took too was Katy Perry's "Firework." It had recently come out while she was going through treatment, and the video features a bald girl with cancer. Emily took it as her personal theme song, and we would play that song over and over again, watching the video. There is something so primitive about music, what it does to our emotions, and how it changes the energy around us. Having positive music fills our rooms with energy. When you're

feeling anxious, calming, meditative music can really quiet your spirit. To this day, if I get a little overanxious, I'll put on a Pandora station of calm meditation music and just let it play, and I'll notice that my breathing slows down. My body slows down. I begin to relax.

Put it into Practice:

- You can get a small wireless speaker to play music in your room.
- Use free stations like Pandora, AccuRadio, or iHeart Radio. You can choose stations based on the type of music you want to play. (tranquil, spiritual, dance, jazz, etc.)
- Make a list of songs that inspire you and create a free playlist of music videos on Youtube. You can then play the entire playlist at once.
- Find songs that your child feels empowered by, ones that focus on strength, courage, bravery, hope, or a positive attitude.

Music Suggestions:

"Your Hands" by JJ Heller

"Good Morning" by Mandisa

"Stronger" by Mandisa

"Roar" by Katy Perry

"Rise" by Katy Perry

"Firework" by Katy Perry

"Go Get It" by Mary Mary

"Mended" by Matthew West

"Rise" by Danny Gokey

"Brave" by Idina Menzel

"Hall of Fame" by The Script

"The Climb" by Miley Cryus

"Fight Song" by Rachel Platten

"I Stand" by Idina Menzel

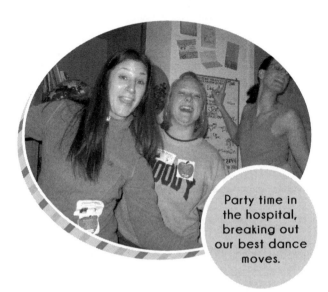

Party time in the hospital, breaking out our best dance moves.

What You See is What You Get

My next step, visualization. At 3 Emily couldn't visualize for herself, so I visualized for her. The doctors said by the end of treatment (those who make it that far) have a 7 out of 10 survival rate. I would picture her being the seventh kid. Over and over, I pictured her older and healthy. Visualizing it and making it real. I could see

that happening. Every time fear would start to creep in, I would close my eyes and picture seven healthy cancer-free kids all lined up, and she was number 7.

Put it into Practice:

- Close your eyes. Picture your child as he or she is now. Now picture them a year from now.
- Begin to imagine, until it seems real, your child growing up.
- Connect with the feelings and sensations in your body as you visualize your child in the future.
- How will you feel the day you walk out of the hospital with your child CANCER-FREE?
- Picture your child 5 years from now:
  - How will he/she look?
  - What will his/her hair look like?
  - What will he/she be doing?
- Picture your child 10 years from now? Ask those same questions.
- Depending on your child's age now, picture the different milestones you will cross.
  - How will you feel watching them start kindergarten?
  - Middle school?
  - High school?
  - Going to the prom?

- Learning to drive? (Now that will be scary!)
- How will you feel watching your Miracle Kid from the audience as he/she graduates high school? Happy and healthy with life ahead of him or her.
- Picture the future. Your child living out his/her dreams, goals, and life's purpose.
- Anytime fear starts to creep in, close your eyes and go back to your visualization making it "feel" as real as possible.

Helpful Hint:

If your child is old enough to understand visualizations you could even do them together. Ask your child what it will feel like as he/she hits these milestones. Have your child close his/her eyes and picture life cancer-free. Fill you child's mind with thoughts and pictures of victory, survivorship, and the future. The mind is a powerful thing. Most of us don't ever come close to utilizing the power of visualization.

ask lots of Questions, But don't Listen to all the answers

I always wanted to know all the possibilities when it came to Emily's treatment. I wanted to know not just all the options, but also all the possible outcomes. Now, I know some people may not want to know some of those outcomes, but for me, I needed to know the worst-case scenario, and the best-case scenario every time. I think because I felt so out of control, knowing the best-case and worst-case gave me that small sense of control. I needed to know exactly what procedures we were doing and what the results were. Then when they told me the best-case and the worst-case, I would always purposely choose to think the best case and then some. Remember, one of the reasons I told Emily she was a Miracle Kid early on was that a Miracle Kid was a kid who did even better than what doctors would expect. So whatever the best, most desired outcome could be, I always thought "and then some." Her outcome would be even better than the best possible outcome. It went back again to, "If there's only a one percent chance, why not be that one percent?"

Put it into Practice:

- Utilize the same skills you've learned with affirmations and visualization.

- Create a positive affirmation for each "best case" scenario.
- Create a mental picture, linked with how you feel, in this "best case" scenario.
- Remind your child he/she is a Miracle Kid and Miracle Kids always do better than the doctors can even begin to imagine.
- Repeat over and over, "If someone's child is going to live, why not mine?" After all, why not?

Patience is Said to Be a Virtue

Practice patience, especially with the staff. I think when we are in crisis mode, in fear mode, it's easy to get angry. Angry at our doctors, angry at our nurses, angry that people aren't doing what we think they should be doing. It was especially difficult for me because I not only had a child with cancer but I also had a restraining order protecting me from her father, who still had visitation rights. We brought with us a long history of domestic violence and abuse, and the hospital wasn't prepared to handle such a complicated family dynamic. It was easy to get frustrated and angry. Particularly when the staff was uneducated and ill-equipped to deal with the dynamics of domestic violence.

It's easy to get frustrated with "the system." Hospitals are run by humans, and humans make mistakes. I am the first one to stand up and say you need to advocate for yourself, and you need to advocate for your child. You need to know all your medicines. You need to know what you're taking. You need to do your research. You can't just blindly trust whatever your doctor will tell you, because you have to remember that they are just human, too. They're just like you and me. Fortunately, I truly believe that the nurses and the doctors who worked with Emily wanted what was best for Emily. Those nurses came day in and day out. They became like family to us. In a lot of ways, the nurses knew my daughter better than the doctors, because they spent the whole day with her. Jocelyn, Melissa, Nanette, Anna, Ann, Erin, the list goes on and on. People who truly gave their heart for Emily. People who wanted what was best for Emily. Who cried when we cried and celebrated when we celebrated. People who, to this day, I am forever grateful for. So, when you're feeling angry and frustrated, take a deep breath and remember, these people have dedicated their lives to saving your child's life.

Put it into Practice:

How to Communicate with the Staff:

- Remember they have lots of patients to attend to. They are doing their best.

- Our kids are our #1 focus, but every kid is their #1 focus.

- Write down questions as you think of them. This will save time later when the doctors or medical experts come by to check in.

- Phrases to use when talking with your medical staff:
  - "What are the other options here?"
  - "Are there any other options or choices?"
  - "If this was your child what would you do?"
  - "Is there anything else I should consider here?"

- If you have a different opinion or want to try an alternative option ask:
  - "Is it reasonable to…"
  - "Would it be possible to try…"
  - If something doesn't make sense, simply say, "I'm not completely understanding. Can you explain that differently?"

Stay Organized:

Put together a "Miracle Kid" notebook. One place you can keep everything together: (A three-ring binder works wells because you can add any discharge papers or medicine pamphlets you might receive.)

- Use your notebook to write down any instructions you are given.
- Use your notebook to keep track of medicines, dosing, or anything else you might need to track.
- You can also keep a section for appointments and names of the various specialists you might be consulting with.
- This is also a great place to write all those questions in!

When a child's spirit is inspired and their heart is healed then the doctors, nurses, and surgeons can come in and do their job. We create the environment to heal their heart, inspire their spirit, and give them that will to fight and live.

You Were Chosen

The more dramatic, silly, and ridiculous we are, the funnier it is to our children. They are so used to seeing us in such serious parental roles that the sillier we are, the more fun it becomes. I think we need to remind ourselves to just have fun. Do we want our kids to remember us as being really serious and sad or just being silly with them? Of course they want the silly!

You know your child best. God entrusted this child to you. There is no better parent for this child than you. Because God chose YOU. Trust your gut. Trust that you are going to do what's best for your child. Trust you know your child's soul, sprit, and heart. You will always know your child's needs. So advocate. Speak up. Speak out. This is all about giving your child the best experience possible. So often I would find that the medical professionals were simply about getting her to the end of treatment. Into remission. They didn't want to talk about long-term effects. They didn't want to talk about long-term consequences. They didn't want to talk about what happened after treatment because the fear was, what if there was no "after treatment?" What if she doesn't make it? We could spend all this time planning out what "after treatment" might look like, but we didn't even know if we were going to get there. We just hope you will have those issues to deal with. We

hope you will have long term effects because it means there is a long-term. For me, from day one, this wasn't just about getting her to the end of treatment but about what life would look like after treatment. What life would look like after cancer treatment wasn't part of our life. What is the big picture? Not just the treatment right here and now but the big picture of how this will affect her emotional well being for the rest of her life. So make it fun!

you can do this!

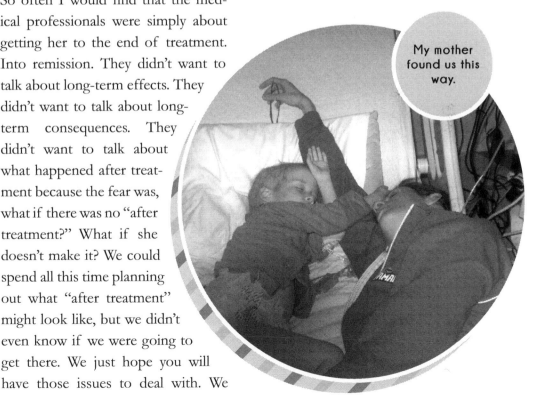

My mother found us this way.

A Peek Into Our World ~ BBA in the B.M.T.

One of the biggest life lessons I have learned in my twelve years in direct sales has been BBA....otherwise known as "Bounce Back Ability." I remember first learning this from National Sales Director Gloria Mayfield Banks, a single mom of two with her MBA from Harvard University. She left corporate America to become a multi-millionaire in Mary Kay, and the #1 person in my division. She shared how a consultant's success in direct sales could be linked to their BBA: how well they "rebounded" from disappointment and setbacks.

How could I ever have imagined a decade ago that lesson, a business lesson, would be put into use during my daughter's fight with cancer. And boy, when I say fight, today it was a fight. Today was the first day I understood what the doctors said when she was first diagnosed: cancer is a roller coaster. An emotional roller coaster you beg to get off and are scared to at the same time, because to get off means defeat. So you stay on...and hold on...and pray.

After checking in with Emily's nurse last night I felt confident she would start her Bone Marrow Transplant process today. We were admitted on Tuesday with plans to start on Wednesday. Everything was going great. She had been home for three weeks going through a series of seventeen tests to prepare for this day. Like everything we do, a party had been planned. We chose a Hawaiian Luau theme. Why? Because it's May, and it's seasonal at the dollar store for Hawaiian Luau party supplies. That's about as creative as I get. She had a cute Hawaiian luau grass skirt and a big fuchsia straw hat. We brought in classic leis for everyone in the hospital, Hawaiian decorations, stickers for her windows, and clings for her wall. Her Secret Stash was packed with luau themed plates, cups, and napkins. She walked into the hospital knowing we were checking in for quite some time. We decorated her room, and we were excited. We gave out leis to every nurse and staff member who was there. We even had a theme song! We choose Miley Cyrus's "Party in the U.S.A." as the perfect theme song for her transplant. We played the song loudly and sang over it just as loudly, "Party in the B.M.T!" While dancing and singing and encouraging everyone else to sing with us. We were having a blast.

Then, at three o'clock, disaster struck in the form of a fever. Two blood draws, one poop scoop, one pee dip, and a handful of sucked up boogers later, everything came back negative. The fever lasted 24 hours and broke. Feeling confident we could begin Friday, we "hung out." Then Thursday afternoon, a delayed test came back positive. Para flu. I had never even heard of Para flu. Now it's become a literal thorn in my side. A respiratory virus. "Virus." The dreaded V word. Nope, it can't be treated with antibiotics; it simply needs to run its course. Your immune system is your only defense. That's nice when your immune system is on a vacation after six rounds of chemo and your lymphocytes are basically nonexistent. I have realized what a disease-infested world we live in and how grateful I am for this little unappreciated thing I have called an immune system. I also now view children as small walking germs and infections...small germ-infested angelic looking faces that are covered with would-be-deadly snot.

However, after having a good weekend with few symptoms, and no fever, we were all counting on a Monday start day. Delayed a week? No big deal. My kid's a rock star. She's a Miracle Baby, remember? Every time she's hit a road block she's overcome it with flying colors...living proof that "Attitude is Everything."

Then morning rolls around. I call. I check in. Really it's just to find out when the chemo's starting. I'm told she is coughing a bit, a little congested. The plan is to discharge her. Here's where medicine is no longer a science. It is an art. Her doctors are the artists, weaving a tapestry of colors that paint a picture of her life...or her death. It's up to them to determine which is a greater risk. Going forward with her B.M.T., wiping out her immune system while she has Para flu, possibly causing it to attack her lungs, cause irreversible damage, and ultimately have her be one the 50% of children who die trying to save their own lives. Or postpone the transplant, wait for it to pass, and pray fervently that her tumor doesn't start to grow during this "incubation period." New growth would mean a complete change in her treatment plan, and her prognosis. I had asked early on when I learned that hers is a tumor that often comes back. "When? When does it come back? What are the "risk times?" Well this is one of those times, the time between her sixth round of chemo and getting her into transplant. I'm scared.

I hang up the phone. I'm on my way to a meeting. My verse, "I know the plans I have for you, declares the Lord, plans to prosper you and not harm you, plans to give you peace and a hope for the future" (Jeremiah 29:11) keeps running through my mind. Google it. Find ten translations. Is there something more in that verse? Some hidden secret maybe I'm missing? Maybe the real translation is, "I know the plans I have for you, declares the Lord, plans to heal your child and perform a miracle and send her home cancer free." Damn can't find that translation. I'm praying as I drive. Lord, please don't take her. And at the same time quietly and guiltily I acknowledge I can't handle the ups and downs of cancer. I wonder, am I the only parent who ever wanted to throw in the towel simply because the not knowing was more painful than the knowing? I weep. Then, as the verse runs through my mind again I remember this same promise God made to me he made to Emily. I imagine God looking down on Emily whispering to her, "I know the plans I have for you...plans to not harm you...a hope for the future." I feel a sense of peace wash over me.

I get to my meeting. My friend Paul asks, "How are you?" as we sit down to eat, and I'm embarrassed I hope he can't see that I am fighting back salty tears that are stinging my eyes. "I'm fine," I say. I tell him briefly what's happening. I won't let my mind go to that negative fearful place. I won't allow those thoughts to manifest in my mind and seep out into the universe where they could travel over interstate 70 and migrate up to the 7th floor and into Emily's room and into her body. We are all connected I remind my mind. My mind will only send her positive belief-filled thoughts. My stomach churns.

Later as I pull into the parking lot at the children's hospital I'm talking to a friend who says how she's so impressed by my positive attitude. She's amazed how I'm holding it together. I tell her it's a choice. I'm choosing to be positive. I'm choosing to declare victory over cancer. I'm "believing it before I see it." Isn't that faith? Hope for what we wish for and certain of what we do not see? (Hebrews 11:1)

I post a Facebook update. As I'm typing I want to type, "Pray she starts BMT." Instead I type, "Pray the safest thing is what happens."

The doctors send her home. I feel defeated. I pull the decorations off her wall. "Why do you have a sad face mommy?" She asks me. "I hate cancer," I respond.

I feel sick. My stomach is in knots, my head is pounding, and I feel physically weak. All the energy has been sucked out of me. We'll have to wait until Friday and they will re-booger test her. If she can't start Monday, everything changes.

As we're leaving the hospital we pass the chapel. Emily wants to stop in to say "Hi" to God. We walk in.

"Hi God, it's Emily Grace. Will you take care of me? Will you stay with me tonight when I sleep? Will you help me do my BMT?" Then she looks at me. "Why is no one else in here she asks? Are they all on precautions? (kids who can't leave their room) Is God going to take care of me?"

"Yes," I say, "He will. I promise."

We get home. I put on Nicole Nordeman. I pray some more. I asked God to have the safest thing happen. She's home. Do I trust that He is keeping her safe? Have I seen Him keep her safe so far? When she was in the ER and the doctors didn't think she should still have been alive? Through her lung surgery, which they didn't know would work? Through her tumor removal, when they said to expect her kidney wouldn't function at least in the beginning? Yes, He has. I will choose to trust Him.

A few hours later it's gone. The fear. This was a setback for sure. Our first cancer wise. Our first disappointment. Our first, "It didn't work the way we planned." Our first BBA. See cancer isn't a physical battle, it's a mental one. I will win. Emily will win. So, if you ever booked a party with me and canceled, or stood me up after I drove to your house in the rain, or didn't return my call after you said you really, really, really wanted to start a Mary Kay business, thank you. Thank you for teaching me BBA. Thank you for teaching me I can't control other people, I can't control cancer, but I can control my attitude. I can sit in the land of self pity and wallow in sadness, despair, and fear. Or I can BB. I can say, "Yup this stinks. I was disappointed. I was hurt. It wasn't what I anticipated. But I'll pick myself up, brush myself off and get back in the game. I'll go to bat again. I'll continue the fight. Cancer, you messed with the wrong mom, I have BBA. You can't keep me down for long." Tonight as I watch Emily sleep, hooked up to her feeding pump, little bald head resting on the pillow, I know every "no" I ever had in business was worth it solely for the fact I have BBA. And she will learn that from me. And if attitude is everything, we're going Jersey Style on this tumor.

* B.M.T. Take 2 ~ The Fairytale. You can imagine the celebration a week later when we checked back into B.M.T. for a second time. Of course, we had already done our Hawaiian luau, so we needed a new theme, and with only one day's notice to plan we didn't have a lot of time. Out of sheer convenience we decided to do a fairy party. Emily already had some cool skirts and fairy wings from other costumes and some wands that people had given her. She also had pink heart sunglasses that matched and sparkly pink shoes that her nurses had given her. For some reason, in addition to her fairy skirt, she wanted me to pin her tiger tail from one of her Halloween costumes onto her fairy outfit. Who knows why she wanted to wear a tail, but later on, when looking at the pictures someone commented, "How cute! A fairy-tail." Some of my favorite pictures, the ones that we've used for most of her posters, are of her in this fairy costume: bald head, pink sunglasses, waving her wand. We went back into the hospital, to party in the B.M.T., and kicked cancer's butt.

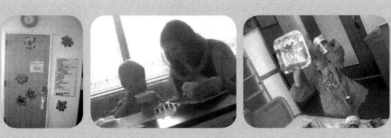

Party in the B.M.T. Take One—Hawaiian Luau Party

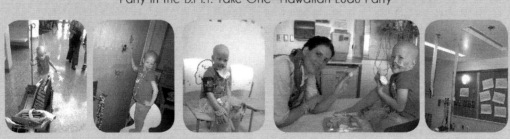

Party in the B.M.T take two—The Fairytale

9 THE ROLLER COASTER CALLED CANCER

It Might Be You That's Nauseous

To say childhood cancer is a roller coaster of emotions is an understatement. Each day, sometimes each hour, can bring with it a flurry of new emotions. A test comes back positive, and we are one step away from instant tears; a test comes back negative, and we are ready to dance through the halls. You're not alone. I think all of us in Club Cancer struggle to navigate the ups and downs that each day, each test, each scan brings. It's enough to make us scream, "STOP! I can't take it anymore!" Our emotional resiliency is pushed to the max. So come hop on the roller coaster of cancer with me and see if you can relate to any of the tips, turns, twists, and twirls we all go through.

is that grief i feel?

Written July 1, 2010

Today Emily was discharged from BMT. It was a day of mixed emotions. Fear, leaving the "safety" and "sterility" of the hospital. The safety of four-hour vitals, twice-a-day doctor checks, and huge PRECAUTION signs outside her door warning everyone to gown up, mask up, and keep germs away from her. In the "real world" no one wears a mask, or a gown, or even comprehends that their small cold, which is no more than a nuisance to them, can be fatal to her.

Yet, it was a day of freedom. With 4th of July almost here, we celebrated a different kind of "Freedom" party today! With red, white, and blue pony tails, hats, ties, and necklaces, we made up a song to celebrate her crossing a major milestone in her cancer treatment. "I'm Free!

> *I never would have made it if I could not have laughed. It lifted me momentarily out of this horrible situation, just enough to make it livable*
>
> Viktor Frankl

I'm Free! I'm bustin' out of B.M.T., woo woo woo!

I'm Free!

I'm Free!

That's right I'm Emily, woo woo woo woo!"

We checked into Brent's place: an apartment-like setting just down the street from the hospital. We will be staying here for awhile.

Emily will stay at this one place, and her father and I will go back and forth. She will be "sheltered" from the outside world, at least temporarily. At our conference with her physician assistant, he advised us to keep her in a "bubble." She can't leave the apartment without her thick blue air filtering mask on. That means she can't eat in public. No picnics and no restaurants. For a mom who's favorite past time is eating out, this was hard to stomach.

"But she loves picnics," I try to explain. "If she is away from crowds and people can she at least lower her mask and take a bite?" I try to negotiate knowing that one of the "goals" Emily had been working so hard for was to leave B.M.T and go on picnics again. The physician assistant looked at me. The first 100 days are the most critical in her recovery. I've heard the stories of kids who breeze through B.M.T only to come back with a yeast or fungal infection. They are deadly. Emily is almost to day 30. "It's 70 days or the rest of her life. I'd err on the side of caution. No picnics." he said. Point taken.

Em sits on the couch not talking. She's mad. This isn't "home." This is a strange apartment. Sterile and unfamiliar. She wants to go home. She's worked so hard to get through her B.M.T. This is her reward?

I know how she feels. I'm unpacking our bags. Trying to put things away. This isn't home. This stinks. I want to be home. In my bed. My kitchen. My stuff. If I feel this way at 33, could I really expect my barely 4-year-old to feel differently.

I bribe her with a "tour" of the place. The game room, the video room, the family area, the playground. She tugs on me. She wants to go outside and play. It's warm. The sun is setting, and it couldn't be a more picturesque time to be outside. I left my phone upstairs. Can I make it through thirty minutes of playing outside without my electric leash? The same kid who hasn't walked further than her hospital bed to the bathroom without crying is now hobbling around the playground. We are the only ones outside. She sits on a green tractor while

I push her around. She checks out the super cool child-size hand-crafted wooden play house, but then decides it has bugs inside and she's outta there. She doesn't talk. Her mask covers most of her face. She points for me to pick up the basketball. She shoots two times and makes both baskets. I'm impressed. Do I have a budding basketball superstar? I would have said she'd be tall enough (I'm 5'10"; her dad's 6'3") but who knows, after radiation she might be short at 5'7". She systematically makes her way through each section of the playground.

As I watch her, I am suddenly overcome with sadness. How many moms take their kids every day to the playground? I know those kids don't appreciate it the way Emily does. Something so normal and mundane to other kids is huge to her. To be outside playing on a playground, hobbling walk and all, is such an exceptional experience for her. I am strangely overcome with this feeling I can't describe. Suddenly it hits me… grief. The realization of how much childhood she has lost because of her cancer.

This will be our eighth month of cancer treatment. In some ways it feels like three. To say eight months sounds so long. Then again, my life BC (before cancer) seems so hard to remember. She has approximately another eight months to go. She'll be almost 5 when she's done. So much time that will just be gone.

I'm grateful for her age. That hopefully she won't remember too much. That she isn't missing her friends, school, and activities. And yet, her pre-school years are so vastly different from other children's. She isn't going to the park, the zoo, or nursery school. She isn't getting to sleep in or play in her home all day. She doesn't go to birthday parties or even get to have a birthday party with other kids. She can't get dirty or play in the pool. She knows words like Broviac, Heparin, and TPN. She draws back her own blood and pukes in the tub. I hate cancer. It's stolen her childhood. It's stolen my precious time with my precious child.

I want her to be "normal." To have to console her because she fell and scraped her knee at the park, not because I just held her down while she screamed, "Mommy make them stop," as a doctor shoved a nose tube down her. I want to cuddle with her and watch a movie and have popcorn and not be in a hospital bed. I want to take her to the Children's Museum, Casa Bonita, and Pirates Cove. I want our days to be ones that don't involve doctor visits, daily temperature checks, and a two-hour bed time routine of line care, feed tubing, fluid pumping, mouth care, and medication. I want to take her to get her pictures done, and to the beach, and to get a kitten. I want to argue with her about staying up past her bedtime not about refusing to take the plate of medicine she needs to swallow every morning.

Today is the first day I feel like I've lost something. Something precious and something I will never recover. I feel guilty. What I have lost is nothing to what Emily has had to go through. I watched her today lying on the radiation table. Her screaming, as she got her fourth nose tube in two months because she keeps puking them up. She screamed, "No! Wait until my med kicks in! Mommy make them wait!" Then she cried, and I cried. Then she screamed, and I closed my eyes and prayed while I held her down.

Yet, it's this moment, watching her on the playground, that makes me sad. I remind myself Emily will be stronger than any kid I know. That she will have an advantage in life simply because she has had to overcome so much at an early age. That God has

plans bigger than I can fathom for her and that her strength and will to fight will serve her the rest of her days. That mastering the "sharing circle" in nursery school is nothing compared to kickin' cancer's butt.

She's standing in front of the big white steering wheel on the playground. She looks at me. Her eyes get wide. She puts her hand to her left ear. She shakes her head and then her butt. "What Em?" I ask. "What do you hear?"

I can't see her face under her mask, but the gleam in her gray/green eyes gives it away. "You hear someone screaming?" I ask. "Someone screaming NO! NO! NO!? Someone who is mad you are on the playground? Is that

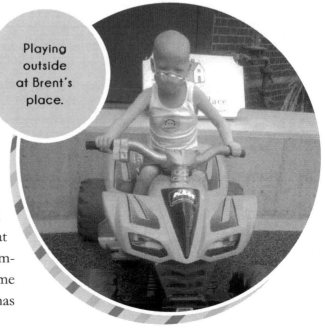

Playing outside at Brent's place.

someone Stupid Tumor?" She nods happily and shakes her head in a "na na na na boo boo" way, nodding in the direction of Stupid Tumor.

It's in that moment I'm reminded of one of my favorite quotes, "The Human spirit is stronger than anything that can happen to it."—C.C. Scott.

I think Emily and I...we'll be okay.

Your Head is a dangerous Place to Be

Monday, Emily had her MRI. The first of three long days of testing to finish her cancer treatment. We've been visualizing, praying, waiting, hoping, and anticipating these three days since she was first diagnosed in November 2009. It seemed so far away at the time, and now it's here. I can barely contain myself. It signifies victory, success, and hopefully the beginning of normal, although I am still not entirely clear what that means anymore.

I can unpack the permanently packed hospital bag full of toiletries, sugar free lemonade packets, and the Bible I took from the hospital chapel in a moment of despair. You are allowed to take them...even in my despair I checked. I will not be scheduling anymore overnight hospital visits, and Emily will only go for checkups now. I always remind people

she is not in remission lest they think they are free to stop praying for her. The next eighteen months are critical. June 2, 2012—that's the date we are waiting for to be in the clear. As for now, we are celebrating her victory for being one of the Miracle Kids that gets to the end of treatment, which increases her cure rate almost 30 percent! What a little warrior she is.

As I'm sitting in the waiting room while she's under anesthesia, a family I know walks by.

"Tara, what are you doing here?" "I'm waiting, Em is having an MRI. We're doing her end-of-treatment scans. Why are you here?"

Then the world stops for a moment. D, their year-old daughter who Em and I saw almost every morning while they did radiation therapy together at University Hospital, has relapsed. She was done; months ago she finished therapy. Her broviac (central implanted IV line) had been removed. She was home. Life was moving on. Then she had an ear ache. Well, it was just an ear ache. Quick trip to the doctor. Except they couldn't see inside her ear. Weird huh? They open behind her ear. There's a mass. It's testing positive for cancer. A blood cancer. But her blood is testing clean. Everyone's stumped. One of the leading cancer doctors in the country can't explain it. Frustration and fear are written all over their faces.

It's a moment like this that reality bites. Cancer kid parents seem to agree. We ache more for each other's kids than our own. Maybe it's because mentally we don't go there with our own kids. We don't face the reality of the fatality of their disease. But when another kid relapses, it triggers that emotional fear…that could be my kid. The pain I feel for this couple. It's empathy to the tenth degree. You've been there too. You know that fear of that first diagnosis. The shock, the grief, the anger, the fight with God. Then the acceptance, the fight, the will to kick cancer's butt. Then victories, infections, trips to the PICU, vomiting, mucositis, narcotic drips, IVS, surgery, tears, clear tests, cheers, success. The inner voice edging you on…she'll be ok…my kid is one of the winning statistic. Then when you hear there is a relapse, everything stops.

Is this worth it? Putting this tiny body through a living hell to gain a year?

I cry for them. I cry for D. I cry for the kids I personally loved and their families that have lost the fight. I am scared and guilty at the same time. Guilty Em is here cancer free, and D is not. Why does my kid get to be the

Miracle Kid? I'm celebrating the end of treatment, and I'm sorry because they are now standing in front of their next mountain. You can just see the tiredness written all over them. Tired of fighting. It's not a physical fight; it's an emotional fight, and some days there just isn't any fight left.

They have to go. I have to go. We say goodbye. I pray for D. God is the only one I know to go to. Then the fear sets in.

I came today in victory. Em is done with treatment. She won! She's my sassy Jersey girl fighter! And now I'm paralyzed in fear. Guilt has suddenly surrounded me. An army of, "What ifs" storm into my brain. What if it's back? What if she's just like the kids I've met who have all lost their battle in the last few months? Children who were the bravest, most heroic cancer warriors who lost. "No!" I scream in my head. I mentally take control of my thoughts and fight back, (once again). I will not let those thoughts take control. I feel sick. The RN comes out. Em's in the Post Op room. (They sedate kids for MRIs).

I go in. I'm trying not to shake. I don't want the hospital staff to think I've suddenly become a junkie on my one-hour break. She's laying there. This tiny little body on a huge operating wheelie bed. Side bars up, a blanket over her, the blue foam head cushion under her. Her eyes are closed, and she is breathing steady. The RN says the MRI went great and confirms they put the catheter in for her next test.

I sit. I think. I try not to think. I stare at her. What if there is cancer in her? What if it has snuck back in and is secretly plotting its human take over? What if all this was for nothing? What if she is just another statistic? She looks so good. Her hair is back and she doesn't have that long yellow spaghetti-like feeding tube sticking out of her nose anymore. She looks...normal. I remind myself for six months she looked normal while cancer was slowly taking over her body and killing her without me knowing. Again, I argue with the fear that torments me. My friend calls to check on Em. I say she's sleeping. Should I tell him? Should I tell him about D and that I'm scared that I want to throw up and run out of here screaming with my hands over my ears. I usually don't tell people I'm scared. I don't want to put that into the universe. Today I do. With my voice shaking I tell him about D, about talking to her family, about her relapse, about my fear.

Now, I know for someone who doesn't live in the cancer world that this is a lot to take in. I barely know what to say to a family when I hear their child has relapsed, and I live it. Can I really expect this poor non-7th floor living, non-chemo puke cleaning, non-hospital eating, sleep room showering, IV pole pushing, CBC reading human to even know what to say? I almost feel guilty for putting him the position of feeling like he has to respond. Should I save him the discomfort? The, "Sorry for your kid, I don't know what to say" moment.

"D isn't Emily."

That's it.

That's all he says.

That's all I need.

He's right. She's not.

Relief literally crashes over like a wave drowning me. I sink into the chair. I feel like I just ran a marathon. "D isn't Emily. D isn't Emily." I repeat it to myself over and over.

I'm sorry for D. I'm sorry for her family. My heart aches for them. I look at Em. She isn't D.

She is cancer-free. She is my Miracle Kid. I won't have the tests back for a few days, and yet suddenly the fear is gone. The fight is back. My Jersey Style kicks in. What was I thinking? FU cancer. You're not taking my kid. She just kicked your butt Jersey style. Get used to it cancer. I might be sitting in Aurora, Colorado, but this is how we do things in Jersey.

cancer kills

It's 2 a.m. I log onto Facebook. I see the post. One of the families I've become close to lost their beautiful daughter to cancer tonight. It had been a really long battle. Reality hits me in the face, and a mental battle starts—a mental battle not to let fear win.

Emily has been doing so well it's easy to "forget" she has cancer. Had cancer. Well, I guess her doctors would say she still "has" cancer. She is still undergoing cancer treatment for six more months. She still is on the "Cancer Kid Roster" and her "Pediatrician" is an oncologist. So I guess technically she "has" cancer. Her last scan was clear. Her last bone marrow aspirate was clear. I tell her she had cancer. She doesn't anymore. Now, we just keep fighting to keep it from coming back.

We've been at home two weeks. It seems like forever. She's playing, laughing, and constantly checking the front window to see if our new neighbors are outside with their two little girls. Kids she can play with. Every day she asks if "the girls" will be outside. Seeing her so desperate for children to play with, my heart aches at her pleas for normalcy.

These are the most "normal" two weeks we've had in almost 10 months. Well, she still won't eat and carries around a canvas bag holding the TPN bag that infuses nutrients into her 12 hours a day—keeping her alive intravenously. But her hair is growing back. She hasn't had an infection in over a month. No more daily temp checks. We're down to just seven meds a day. I've gotten used to the, "Whats?" as we wait on her hearing aids. It's so easy to think we are in the clear.

And then I read a post at 2 a.m. Another child has died. That's the fourth in the span of just a few months. And those are only the ones I know. Another beautiful child who fought and fought and lived the last year of her life in a hospital bed lost her battle. A family that prayed, cried, and kept a positive attitude. A mother who lost the baby that she once held in her arms and imagined her future and who she would become.

Reality slaps me in the face at 2 a.m. The scans may be clean, but my child has cancer. Cancer kills. Cancer takes dreams and goals and futures without bias. Cancer kills children. Children who fight and win the battles only to lose the war. If the devil created a disease, cancer would be it. It quietly kills your spirit before it kills your body. Cancer. I have emotionally detached myself from the word. Remember, I am careful about what I say and what words I give power to. "Emily is undergoing cancer treatment." "Emily had a tumor." "Emily's scans are clear of cancer." "Emily will be a person who had cancer." Emily. My child. The only saving grace from an eight-year abusive marriage. The child who gave me the will to keep going when I was so deep in depression at the end of my marriage that I didn't care about anything, even getting out of bed. Emily, the child who was my reason for putting one foot in front of the other when my world collapsed. The child who each day gives me a reason to not give up.

I climb into the toddler bed with her to just hold her and to listen to her sleep. Tears stream, and I ask God to forgive me for the moments I get frustrated with her and don't appreciate every second I have with her. This past week flashes before me.

Getting frustrated that it was 10 p.m. and she still wouldn't go to sleep. That every time I left the room she'd start crying and get of bed.

"Em, I told you I was going downstairs to check on my bagel." ~ " BUT I MISSED YOU!"

"Em, I told you I was going to the bathroom." ~ "BUT I NEED YOU!" "Em, I told you I was going to brush my teeth." ~ "BUT I COULDN'T SEE YOU!"

"Em, I told you I was going to wash my face" ~ "BUT I DIDN'T WANT YOU TO!"

"Em, I told you not to get out of bed!" ~ "BUT I HAD TO!"

Then the millionth time she said, "Mommy??!!???" and I said, "Em just stop! Don't ask me another question!"

And then, finally, when I said, "Em, I'm beat. I'm going to bed."

And she asked. "Mommy what if I need to puke, can I call you?"

"Yes, Em."

"Will you wake up and hear me?"

"Yes, Em."

"Will you come get me?"

"Yes, Em."

"Will you get a me a puke bucket?"

"Yes, Em, just go to sleep!"

"Mommy?"

"Yes Em?" with mounting exasperation.

"Will you get me a tissue to wipe my face if I puke?"

"No, Em just use your sheets!"

But now it's 2 a.m. I'm overcome with guilt and begging God to forgive me for not being grateful I was tucking her into her own bed and not a hospital bed.

Forgive me God.

I'm sorry for every time I resent having to get four syringes, two needles, two vitamin vials, blue connectors, saline, a pump, a new battery, tubing that I can never get to connect properly and end up screaming at and wanting to throw across the room, a giant bag of TPN and more alcohol prep pads than I can count.   Instead of being grateful that science has created a way to keep my child alive while her stomach has shrunk so small that when she doesn't eat she gets a hunger pain and when she does eat she still gets pain because her stomach has literally "forgotten" how to eat.

I'm sorry for every time I have to change a diaper, and I'm mad she isn't potty trained anymore after spending almost nine months in a hospital bed. Instead of being grateful that pee and poop aren't blood and vomit.

I'm sorry I resent that I can't take her out to eat, go to Pirate's Cove (because yes, I want to go), go to outdoor summer music concerts (because yes, I want to go), or go on a picnic (still me who wants to go). Instead of being grateful I can sit

on the couch, cuddle her, and read her a book.

I'm sorry I resent watching my checking account dwindle from the cost of gas and having to drive back and forth to the hospital multiple times each week. Or the swipe, swipe of my debit card from all the meals I've had to buy at the hospital while we are there. Instead of being grateful I can drive back and forth and that I have a car to drive, instead of being like the families I see outside the hospital waiting for the bus, grateful I have money and people who've helped with gas, and that going back and forth means she's winning her battle and isn't in the PICU dying.

I'm sorry I resent seeing piles and piles of toys scattered all over my family room. I remind myself of my vow that I will be grateful for those bags of toys, because toys mean Emily's home with me.

I'm sorry I resent I turned down three dates in two weeks because I had her with me, and I secretly dream of a "normal life" too. Instead of being grateful that she is my life, because without her my life would never be "normal" again.

I'm sorry that as we get closer to the end of treatment I start "planning" again. Setting goals for work and worrying about how I'll manage Emily and working full time again. Instead of appreciating that I get to juggle work and Em, that daycare isn't part of that plan, and that she is finally old enough to go with me for almost everything. Reminding myself that school is just around the corner, and I need to appreciate this short precious time when she is with me before friends, sports, and homework take over.

I'm sorry there is a part of me that dreads packing my suitcase this week to have to live back at the hospital. Instead of being grateful that biotherapy is available to Emily. Because it only became available nationally just over a year ago and increases her cure rate by 15%-20%.

I kiss her peach fuzz head. Her hair is growing back dark. The click click of her pump echoes in the dark. I'm grateful that at 5'10" I'm still small enough to fit in her toddler bed with her. I savor this moment just holding her. I can't imagine my life without her. Without her constant barricade of questions, "Mommy!" fits, demands, and giggles.

I lay there in a mental war. Fear is attacking every corner of my mind. The four kids who have recently died. Their names, their faces, and their parents' faces flash in my mind. Cancel. Cancel. I fight back. The colors of life death sign flashes past me. "Cancel," I say. A picture of my life without Em fights to gain a foothold in my mind. Cancel. Cancel. I refuse to let fear win. After biotherapy, statistically 6.5 to 7 out of 10 children will never relapse. They will go on to live their lives cancer-free. Since you can't have half a kid I round up to seven. 7 out of 10. Then there are kids who never make it to biotherapy. I remind myself of Emily's Bone Marrow Conference. Her doctor, standing at the board going over her next level of therapy and saying, "If she makes it to biotherapy..." I remember screaming at him in my head, "YES! She will make it! There is no IF!" And she has. She is one of those kids. If seven out of ten make, it why not her? I picture seven healthy cancer-free kids in my mind. I picture Emily as one of the seven. Repeating my mantra, "Why not? Why not her?" If someone has to be the statistical seven, why not Emily? She is, after all, my Miracle Kid.

The next morning Emily wakes up and asks me when she goes back to the hospital.

"Tomorrow." I tell her. "We have to plan your party!" I say trying to make it fun. You can see the look of sadness come over her face. She knows what going to the hospital for a week will mean.

"It will be great, Em. We can see Nanette, Melissa, Jocelyn, and Anna, all your faves." She agrees. Life seems strange without these women, these nurses, who have become our family this year.

"And Emily," I say and hold up five fingers, "When you are done with this week, you have just four more to do. Then you're done with cancer!"

She peers at me and smiles, "Then I can have a normal life?" she asks.

"Well, still checkups, but that's it."

"Yup, just checkups." I respond.

"Mommy, will you hold my hand when I have to get the finger poke?" (She knows that checkups mean her broviac implant comes out and then her blood draws will be "finger pokes.")

"Yes, Em, I'll hold your hand."

"Okay, Mom," and she snuggles back in.

She reminds me that even after treatment, cancer will always be part of her life.

We will never be "cancer-free."

Those regular checks ups will be constant reminders of her strength, her will, her victory...and my gratefulness.

Emily Has Eyelashes

It's funny how something so "normal" seems to strange. I have gotten so used to seeing her without hair that the short rim of dark lashes around her gray/green eyes looks odd.

I remember when her hair first fell out. These crazy Shirley Temple curls were her "signature." Everywhere we went people would comment on her hair. I remember the first night they transferred us from the PICU up to the "bear" floor. I was walking down the hall with my cousin and a teenager was walking in front of us who was completely bald. I remember that tight feeling in my chest. A stark slap of reality. I am on a cancer floor. I have a child with cancer. I will be the mom of a baldy.

That night as she sat on my lap, I took sharp orange scissors and cropped her hair close to her head. I cried. I tried not to. I didn't want her to cry too. She didn't. I put a thick piece of curls in a lab bag. I wanted to save it. The nurses told me her hair, when it grew back, might grow in differently. I wanted to remember what my daughter was before she was a cancer kid, when she was innocent and naive to the medical world.

Now, fast forward nine months. I am so used to seeing her without hair I am not sure how to react to the small patches that are slowly growing back on her head. She has short dark eyelashes and tufts of eyebrow patches.

There was a brief time before her transplant when her hair had started to grow back in a dark buzz evenly and all over her head. It was different then. It only lasted a few days, and I knew it was going to fall out again as I watched the chemo drip into her over ninety-six hours. This time, though, the hair will stay. There is no more chemo. It's done. She has one day left of radiation, and then that's done too. Her hair will grow back, and she will look normal again. Her bald head is a badge of courage everywhere she goes. She doesn't wear hats or scarves or anything. She loves her bald head and keeps reminding me as I check out the new patchy hair growth that she will be shaving it off as soon as it grows back.

Right now, she has the same hair as a little old man. Lots of hair in a horseshoe around the back of her head and a two-inch tuft off the top. I have asked the doctors three times if it will all grow in or are these bald patches permanent? They keep assuring me it will just grow in at different times but eventually will all grow in. I'm not convinced yet.

At the same time, I have to admit her hair growing back scares me. It's a reminder that chemo is over and we are onto the next part of her therapy.

Biotherapy. I just had the consult with her doctors today, and I have the consent forms sitting in my bag to sign and bring back in on Tuesday. Biotherapy (also known as immune therapy) lasts six months with five treatments. She'll go into the hospital on a Monday and stay the week. She'll check out Friday and then have a three-week break. She'll only need to come back to the clinic one time the following week, and then only if she is sick. The kids usually do great at home, and after September 9, her 100th day past post bone marrow transplant, her mask comes off and she can start to resume a normal life.

Biotherapy is hard. It's painful. Really painful. The kids are put on a narcotic drip upon admission. Two of the five rounds are done in the PICU from the beginning (because so many kids end up being transferred, they just start them there now). Em will be the third kid at this hospital getting this particular round of therapy. It's not FDA approved yet. Kids who make it all the way through increase their long-term survival rate 15-20%.

I am told they will do whatever they have to do to keep her alive to get the drugs into her. Blood pressure meds, ventilators, ART lines: it's a race against time. The medicine goes in over ten hours. If she starts to react they slow it down. It has to be in within twenty hours. Whatever doesn't make it in within the twenty hours is discarded and you start over the next day. Obviously, the more that goes in the higher her cure rate. I sign a fourteen page consent packet. Pages of side effects. All scary. A relapse scarier. I sign away.

I should be excited her hair is growing back. It means the end of chemo. I'm not. I know chemo. It's comfortable. I know what to expect. Biotherapy is scary. It's new territory. The unknown. And then, when it's over...you wait. The scariest part of all. You scan. You wait. You scan. You wait. You try to live without fear and you cherish life in a way most people will never understand. I guess it's a choice to be grateful or resentful. I'm not sure which choice I'll make yet.

Those dark patches of hair represent the "real world." Shampoo, haircuts, and bows. They are all part of the real world. Washing your 4-year-old's head with a wash cloth? That is not. My reality is skewed. The real world lies outside the four walls of a hospital room. The real world, where dealing with life right now actually feels more overwhelming than dealing with cancer. Here, the nurses are

our family. The cafeteria my kitchen. The parking lot my garage. It's my life. Hair...that's not my life.

I look at her dark patchy tufts of hair. I wonder what she will look like. The bald child I see now is not the one I brought to the emergency room almost a year ago. That child didn't have nightmares of getting poked. That child didn't have yellow tinged bruises on her legs that never seem to fully go away from week after week of insulfon needles being placed. That child didn't have a "diamond cut" scar across her belly or holes in her side where chest tubes stayed for months. That child didn't know how to draw her own blood back out of a central line implanted in her chest or know that when she is "pukey" she wants Ativan and when she is in pain she wants Oxycodone. That child didn't know the difference between an X-ray, a CAT scan, and a MIBG scan. That child didn't say, "What? What?" all the time and didn't need hearing aids. That child had hair.

I will miss kissing her bald head. I will miss the visible reminder that Emily is different. Her bald head represents her strength to me. Her will to win. Her courage. Hair will make her like every other kid. As strange as it sounds, I'm glad she's not. I'm glad she's a fighter. I'm glad she's got a "reputation" for being strong willed and for being the only 3-year-old to pull out her own chest tube. I'm glad she is young enough to hopefully not remember the bad parts and old enough to remember she is a Miracle Kid and she can do anything. I wonder how having cancer will mold who she will become. How it will shape her destiny in a way that having hair never would have. Because, even after her hair grows back…however it grows back, light, dark, straight, or curly… she will always be my brave, beautiful, bald kid.

Reality…here we come.

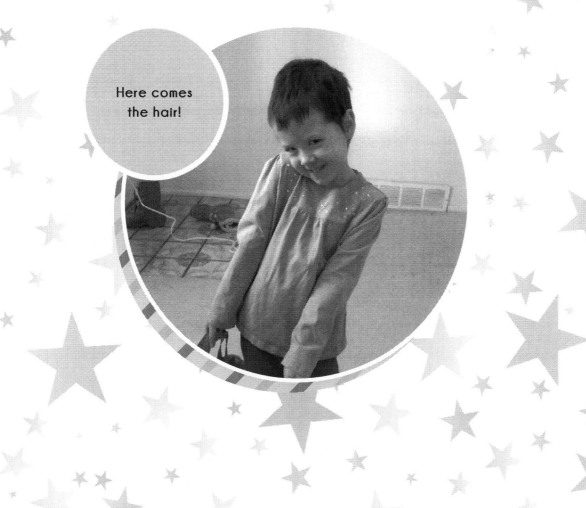

Here comes the hair!

the ROLLER COASTER is not FUN. STePS FOR STepping Off:

Let's be honest. We can't get off the roller coaster. But maybe there's a way to at least handle the drops and turns a little better. Think of it as the parent's version of Zofran, it helps alleviate the nausea!

What is the hardest part of being the parent of a Miracle Kid? _____

_____

_____

_____

What are the major emotions you find yourself experiencing daily?

Sadness	Loss of Control	Love	Anger	Grumpiness
Terror	Disgust	Anxiety	Grief	Calmness
Dread	Courage	Anguish	Isolation	Shame
Regret	Optimism	Hatred	Panic	Frustration
Pity	Exasperation	Nervousness	Loneliness	Hostility
Annoyance	Envy	Helplessness	Compassion	Hope
Jealously	Pain	Grouchiness	Homesickness	Worry
Rage	Pride	Indignation	Sorrow	Aggravation
Fear	Impatience	Sulkiness	Determination	Acceptance
Irritation	Bitterness	Resentment	Resolve	Happiness

Resignation (giving up)

What do you wish other people knew about what you are going through? _____

_____

_____

_____

_____

Who are two people you feel comfortable talking to?

1. _____

2. _____

What would you want to say to them?

_____

_____

_____

_____

What would you like them to say back to you?_____

_____

_____

_____

_____

How would this help?_____

_____

_____

_____

_____

Are you willing to share both what you want to say AND how you are hoping they will respond? (Remember most people want to help but have no idea what to say or do!)

_____

_____

_____

_____

FINDING SUPPORT

- Does the hospital have a support group for parents?
- If not, do they have any recommendations for one?
- Does your hospital have a social worker? Someone you can talk to?
- Will your insurance cover personal counseling or therapy?
- Does your church or religious organization offer counseling or support groups?
- Is there a parent "post cancer" that would be willing to talk to you?
- Look online, there are lots of groups popping all the time. Momcology (www.momcology.org) and American Childhood Cancer Organization (www.acco.org) are good places to start.

You don't need to go through this alone. Remember our stats on Club Cancer from Chapter 1? There are lots of parents going through the same roller coaster of feelings. I probably felt every feeling on that list at one point! Don't suffer alone. Ask for help.

10

HOW LONG IS LONG ENOUGH?

Me, God, and the Bathroom Floor

I'm sitting on the bathroom floor, back against the door paralyzed in fear. My head down, my hands pressed together, and tears streaming down my face. I just got off the phone with my mother. Crying, because I saw a spot. Emily has just completed three days of testing. Having her "end of treatment scan" to make sure she has remained cancer free now that therapy is ending. We've been looking forward to this day all month. End of therapy. What will that mean? It sounds exciting. It feels like jumping off a bridge into an abyss where life can start again and be somewhat normal.

As she laid there during her scan, and I jumped around her room to make it fun, I glanced over to the testing screen and saw a spot. Not just one spot, but a number of spots. Dark black patches on her X-rayed body. There on the screen. Fear washed over me like a tidal wave. I couldn't let Emily know. I started shaking. Using every acting technique I ever learned in college not to let my Miracle Kid see my pending panic attack. The test finished and I distracted her to talk to her tech.

"What the heck is that on the screen???!!!"

"Tara, you can't look at this," she says.

Is that a look of fear I see in her eyes? Legally, she can't say anything to me.

"Do you have an appointment today with her oncologist?" she asks.

I nod my head yes. "You have to talk to her," the tech responds.

I look at the screen. I've seen enough screens to know this looks wrong. Really wrong.

I barely remember the drive home. I put on a fake "everything is great" voice and brought Emily upstairs to bed for a nap. She was tired. I tuck her in and kiss her head. I can't let her see my paralyzing fear. I'm fighting every scary

> **Always find a reason to laugh, it may not add years to your life but it will add life to your years.**
>
> Unknown

thought attacking my brain right now. I call my mom. She tells me to wait until I talk to the doctor. I know she can't tell me she's now terrified too. Just like I have to be brave for my daughter, she has to be brave for me. I hang up.

I'm now locked in my bathroom, kneeling on the floor, screaming to God. Not sure why I think God is in the bathroom, but that's where I am. "I need to know!" I cry out. I need to know if she is going to die. I know that at this point if her cancer has returned, treatment is about prolonging life not a cure. I can't take it anymore. Months after months of an emotional roller coaster. Waiting for lab work, scans, urine tests, and X-ray results. Just days ago with D during her MRI. I am at my end. The stress has taken its toll. I will deal with whatever happens, but I just need to know if she lives or dies. I beg God for an answer. I tell Him I am refusing to leave this bathroom until I have an answer. Like Honi the Jewish prophet who drew a circle in the sand and refused to move until God sent the rain, I am not moving until I know. I demand to know.

I don't know how long I stayed in that bathroom but when God answered me; His answer was loud and clear. With a little "how dare you demand me" attitude mixed in.

"How long is enough? How long does Emily need to live for YOU to feel you beat cancer? What if she makes it till 7 and is in remission and then at 18 dies in a car accident? Will you feel you have won? What if she beats cancer and dies from an aneurysm in her sleep at 30? Will you be satisfied? What if at 50 she drops dead of a stroke? Will you think that was long enough? How long do you, little human, think "long enough" is? Don't you realize long enough will never be long enough? I am her Father in heaven. She is my child first. You are just her mother here on Earth and you will have her as long as I give her to you. Don't take any day for granted. And remember, no matter what happens, I will still be here for you."

I get up. God's right. Anytime a child dies before a parent there is insurmountable grief. No matter what the cause. I have the fear of cancer now, but there will be other fears as she gets older. The first time she gets behind a driver's seat and drives away in a car. Later praying she never gets in a car with a drunk driver. When she goes off to college alone or chooses to fly across the world. Will I ever not worry about her? Just because she doesn't have cancer doesn't mean something else can't kill her. People lose their children every day, and it's not to cancer. Grief is grief, no matter the cause. No matter what happens with these scans, no matter what happens in life, I will get through it. Because I am strong, and I have chosen to trust God even when I don't agree with Him.

I dry off my tears. I wait for the doctor's call. I pick up and simply say, "I know, I saw the scans." The doctor has no idea what I am talking about. Emily's scans are clear, and she remains cancer free. That can't be true, I argue, (because clearly my theater training background has equipped me to read a scan better than a trained radiologist). Her oncologist believes maybe I saw her organs, or it might have been a variation in the pictures (they can adjust them lighter or darker), but there definitely was no cancer. Congratulations, Emily is done.

I hang up. The energy has literally drained out of me, and I feel empty. Was I wrong, or was it a miracle?

Honestly, to this day, I don't know. What I do know is that day changed me forever. I know no matter what happens, ever, in life I will be okay. I will trust God, trust that He loves my Miracle Kid even more than I do. I will never take one day with my child for granted. When she is done with her purpose here on Earth He will take her back. And in the end, each of us wakes up each morning one day closer to dying.

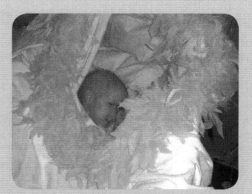

Some days your just hide from the world.

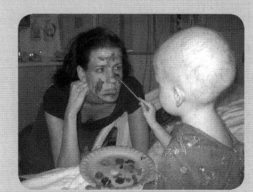

MCF painting mommy's face.

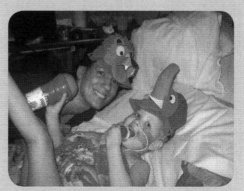

Silly hats make every day fun.

WHAT I LEARNED FROM MY MIRACLE KID

- You're stronger than you think.
- Nothing lasts forever.
- You can do anything for a short time.
- It really is all about attitude.
- The mind is a powerful thing; it remembers what it wants.
- Every day we have a choice.
- Giggles are contagious.
- There's no such thing as too silly.
- You can be happy even lying in a pile of pickle puke.
- Nothing replaces friends, family, and people in your life who care about you.
- What you give to others really does come back to you.
- Work when you can; you never know when you can't.
- Sometimes the morally right thing isn't always the right thing.
- The most important decision you will ever make in your life is who you marry.
- When it comes to your kids, you can really be superhuman. Having to flush vials, having to do the nose tube; things that I never thought I could do, I do.
- Trust yourself; you know your body, your mind, and your spirit best.
- There's nothing more powerful than love. The way I feel about Emily, the love for a child, truly there's nothing more powerful. It allows us to do incredible things. To move mountains. To make the impossible possible. To go days without sleep, nights without rest, and still function.
- Never, ever, envy someone else's life. You have no idea what the future holds.
- Perspective is the most interesting gift. Stop and think about perspective. It can always get worse, be grateful for what you have. I remember driving down Interstate 470, wishing I could go back to just my divorce when life was scary but manageable.
- Forrest Gump was right, "Life truly is like a box of chocolates; you really don't know what you're going to get."
- Life is precious; believe it. It can change in an instant.
- Milk and Oreos can fix just about anything.
- Sometimes you need to be good to yourself. Sometimes you need to give yourself a break.
- You have a voice, share it.

WHaT i'M LeaRNiNG FROM MY MiRacLe Kid

- _____
- _____
- _____
- _____
- _____
- _____
- _____
- _____
- _____
- _____
- _____
- _____
- _____
- _____
- _____
- _____
- _____
- _____
- _____

11

THE CONCLUSION
But Not the End

Just when I've fallen back into the BC me, it's time again for scans. As I write this, our bi-annual scans are just days away. Those scans every few months seem like God's reminder for me to put things in perspective. It's that one tie that keeps us connected back in the cancer world where nervousness, anxiety, and fear live. It's the reminder of the little voice asking you, "What are you really stressing out about? Look at what's really important. Stop and appreciate the people who are around you. Life can change in an instant. Overnight. In one car trip. One hospital visit. Or one bad bug. What are you getting upset about? Just appreciate. Be grateful."

So how do I find that balance? How do any of us? Not staying in the cancer world but staying in a place of total appreciation of every single moment. Staying in a place where I'm able to evaluate what truly is important, what truly is worth stressing over and what's not. Remembering, all of this is fleeting. And not only is it fleeting, it is quickly fleeting. It will be over in an instant. All of us have that date coming. The day that we leave this Earth and return to our Father in heaven. We don't know when, but I think we will all feel it came too quickly. So it's our choice. Time is a gift we have been given. It's our conscious decision to choose how we use the time we have now, today, and in this moment. Cancer will not choose; I will choose. Will we live in fear, in worry, in anger? Or will we choose something different? Choose to live in joy, peace, gratitude, love, and fun? For me, I will choose the latter. In the end that is all any of us really have control over anyway.

> The world is round and the place which may seem like the end may also be only the beginning.
>
> *Ivy Baker Priest*

I don't know if the fear of those scans will ever go away. I don't know if those little dark thoughts that try to creep into my head every now and then, will ever be silenced permanently. I do know that every time I start to think those thoughts, in my head I say "cancel," and I picture Emily, a healthy, strong little girl, young adult, and grown woman.

Sometimes it's hard not to feel like a victim of our circumstance; I feel life robbed us of those years. Life robbed my daughter of a childhood, of a preschooler, of a 3-, 4- and 5-year-old life. It took away her innocence, and it took away mine.

However, it also gave us a new perspective. It gave me appreciation for life and those little moments in a way I never had before. All parents celebrate their child's birthday, but when you celebrate the birthday of a child who had cancer, well that's a whole different kind of celebration. It truly is a celebration of life. There are still moments when, all of a sudden, I will be overwhelmed with gratefulness, and I will suddenly break down crying. Grateful for those moments with her. Sometimes it's hard; those long-term effects don't go away. Every time she has to get a hearing test, I'm reminded she'll never hear the same way again. Every time we go in for a scan or even just a basic trip to the pediatrician, she's angry, she doesn't want a poke, she doesn't want a shot, and I'm reminded she's not like other kids. Every time she has a temper tantrum or separation anxiety, or fear of something unknown, something new that's going to happen, I have to remind myself that her experience

and the way she's viewed the world and experienced the world is different than how most children have. It's different from my childhood. She's lost her innocence in a lot of ways. The world can sometimes feel really scary for her and she'll act out. Walking that fine line as a parent, between making excuses, versus acknowledging what they've gone through. I don't want Emily to be constantly known as the kid who had cancer. I don't want her to constantly get exceptions or excuses because, "Oh, she had cancer."

Yet, at the same time, she did have cancer. It does shape who she is, how she acts, and what she has to do. I think that will always be a tightrope her whole life. The guilt as a parent for knowing what your child's been through and at the same time not letting them use that as an excuse to not be their best.

I don't know if there's a right way to do it; I don't even know if there's even one way to do it. Each of us on this journey takes a step forward, then takes a step back. Takes a step forward, then takes a step sideways. Tries something new.

Each child, circumstance, and experience is different. We're different. I don't think any two parents can have the same experience, or the same outcome. It changes our world, and it shapes who we are. Some of us lose our children along the way, we lose the battle, and our lives are forever changed. Some of us don't lose our children. We feel grateful and guilty.

As we get further and further removed from the cancer world, it's easy to fall back into "the real world," life, stress, getting upset over small things…getting frustrated in traffic, getting annoyed when there are toys on the floor, getting overwhelmed with laundry, grocery shopping, to-do lists. Life goes on, and you go back to the daily stresses. It's easy to forget. I never thought I would. I never thought I would let the small stuff get to me again. As time goes on, I'm finding I do get stressed out about insignificant things again. I get frustrated. I lose my patience. I feel jealousy, anger, and resentment. I didn't experience those in the hospital. I was so grateful for the tiny little victories. Some of us want to run: we want to hide, and pretend that that part of our life is over. Once we're out of treatment, we want it to be in the past, never having to experience it again. I know. I felt that way. I believed that part of my life was over. I'm moving on, and I want to forget all the horror that went along with it.

I don't know how long Emily will live. I hope it's a long time. I pray it's a long time. I know after my day on the bathroom floor, I've turned it over to God. I have decided that no matter what happens, I will trust Him. I have decided I will be grateful for every second, every moment, every hour, every week, every month, and every year. I will continue to pray for many, many years. I hope that Emily's cancer experience shapes her into a strong, powerful, confident adult. I hope that as she faces life, she's reminded of what a warrior she is. How strong she is. I hope that she always considers herself a Miracle Kid. I hope when faced with things or people who say, "You can't do this," that she can look them squarely in the eye and say, "I beat cancer at three. Don't tell me what I can't do." I hope that some of the trauma, fear and anxiety will slowly fade away and turn into willpower, determination, courage, and bravery, character traits that will take her far. I hope she doesn't let cancer define her, but that it becomes defining. That she won't always see herself as a kid who had cancer, but she will always see herself as someone who kicked cancer's butt. That she will see herself as somebody strong, who faced death in the eye courageously and boldly and now can do anything. She truly is the bravest person I have ever met. Sometimes I feel so inadequate to be her mom. How could God have trusted me with the bravest person in the world? What a responsibility I have to raise her. And while it's a privilege, I'm also aware of that incredible responsibility. I believe God kept her alive for a reason. I wonder what that reason is. I can't wait to see what kind of beautiful woman she grows up to be, what she'll do with her life, and what gifts and talents she'll contribute to the world. I pray that she will leave her mark in a big way. I often think she must. How could she not after everything she's been through? How could she not have a powerful presence? A powerful story to leave a powerful mark.

Often it is said, you need to let go of your story to move out of the past and into the future. There's talk about victims going back to their "story" over and over again. While I see the value of leaving our past behind, in many ways, our stories shape who we are. They shape how we see the world, and our future, and Emily's cancer story is part of our life now. It doesn't go away simply because we move into the future. It's

changed us; it's changed our spirit; it's changed our heart; it's changed us, permanently. We can either have this change be positive or negative. We can constantly go back to how unfair life is, how much we had to give up and sacrifice, and certainly there are moments where I struggle with anger, remorse, and sadness.

Sadness that I will never get to have the childhood experience with her that I wanted. Regret; could I have done things differently? Did I make all the right medical choices for her? There's a whole mishmash of feelings that can sweep over experiencing ten different feelings in what seems like less than a minute. That story, Emily's story, it's her story. It's what she will bring into her future and choose to define who she is. It's what she's going to do with her story that will make a difference. It's how she will use her story to remind herself how strong she is, how courageous she is, how brave she is, and how she really can get through anything. Our stories are what make us strong. Our stories are what build our spirits. This is Emily's story.

ABOUT THE AUTHOR

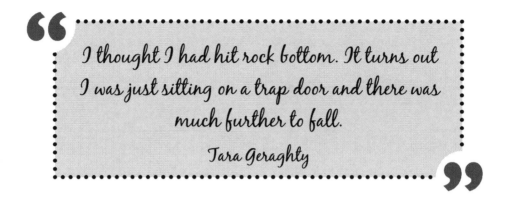

> " *I thought I had hit rock bottom. It turns out I was just sitting on a trap door and there was much further to fall.*
>
> *Tara Geraghty* "

Tara has spent over 20 years in leadership development. She holds a degree in theater and has a background in improvisation. It was those three unlikely skill sets which she drew upon in 2009 when her 3-year-old daughter was diagnosed with high risk stage 4 neuroblastoma. She choose to face cancer with fun, and to support her daughter in a non-traditional way. Tara now shares those powerful tools, tips, and secrets to help parents navigate the scary world that is childhood cancer. Tara is the author of Making Cancer Fun: A Parents Guide, I'm a Miracle Kid workbook, From Living to Being, The Rock Star Calendar and the creator of the The Grateful Connection Course. She is a contributing author on Every Entrepreneur's Guide to Running your Own Business, a regular contributor to Conquer Magazine: The Patient's Voice, and can be heard on podcasts worldwide. She lives in New Jersey with her miracle kid Emily Grace and their chiweenie.

Made in the USA
Middletown, DE
20 March 2019